Getting Ready for My **Hernia** Surgery

Hernia Surgery Book for Kids - Preparation and Recovery

This book belongs to:

Written by Dr. Fei Zheng-Ward   Illustrated by Moch. Fajar Shobaru

Copyright © 2025 Fei Zheng-Ward

All rights reserved. Published by Fei Zheng-Ward, an imprint of FZWbooks. No part of this book may be copied, reproduced, recorded, transmitted, or stored by any means or in any form, electronic or mechanical, without obtaining prior written permission from the copyright owner.

Identifiers: ISBN 979-8-89318-125-8 (eBook)
　　　　　　 ISBN 979-8-89318-126-5 (paperback)
　　　　　　 ISBN 979-8-89318-127-2 (hardcover)

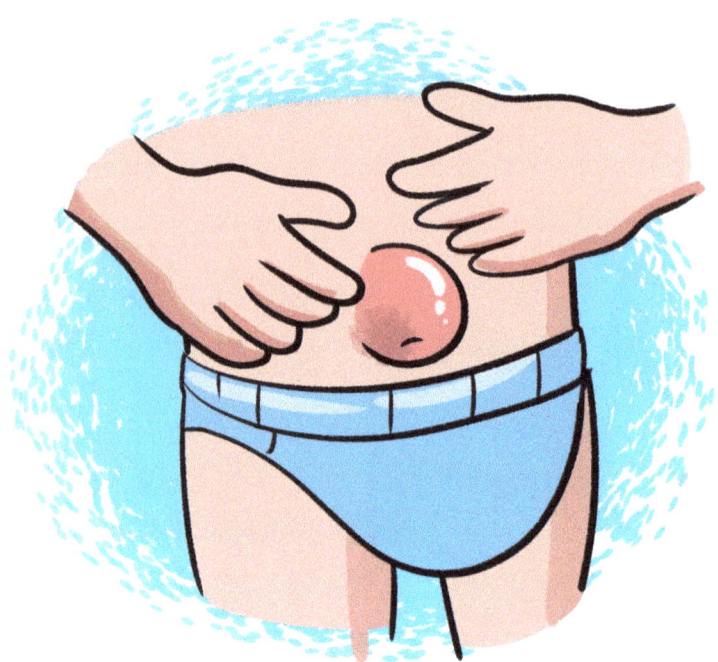

A hernia happens when something soft inside your tummy pushes through a thin spot in the wall of your belly. This makes a little bump under your skin.

Think of it like blowing a bubble with gum. If the gum has a thin spot, the air pushes through and makes a bubble.

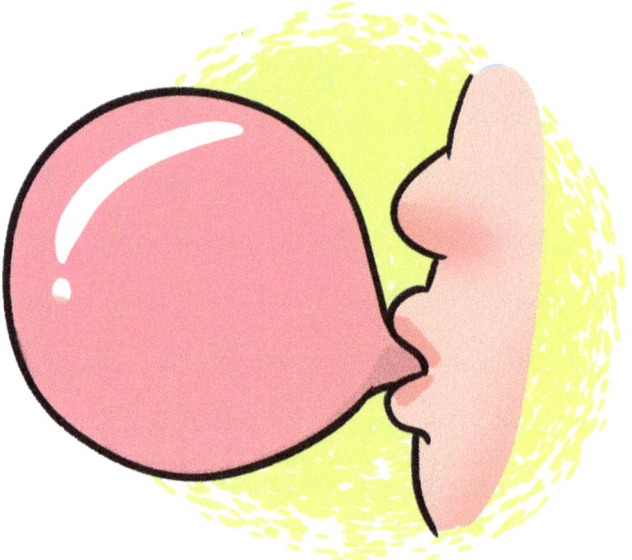

What is a hernia?

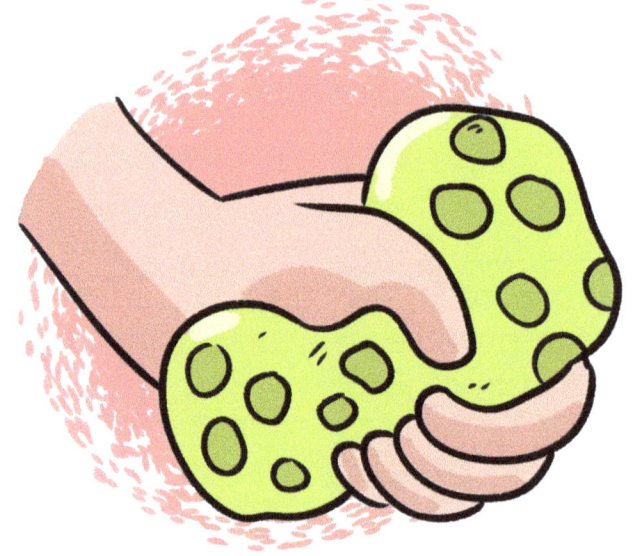

Or like squeezing a squishy stress ball filled with little beads. Some beads can poke out through the thin spots of the ball.
That's kind of what happens with a hernia.

The bump may get bigger when you cough, sneeze, cry, or lift heavy things.

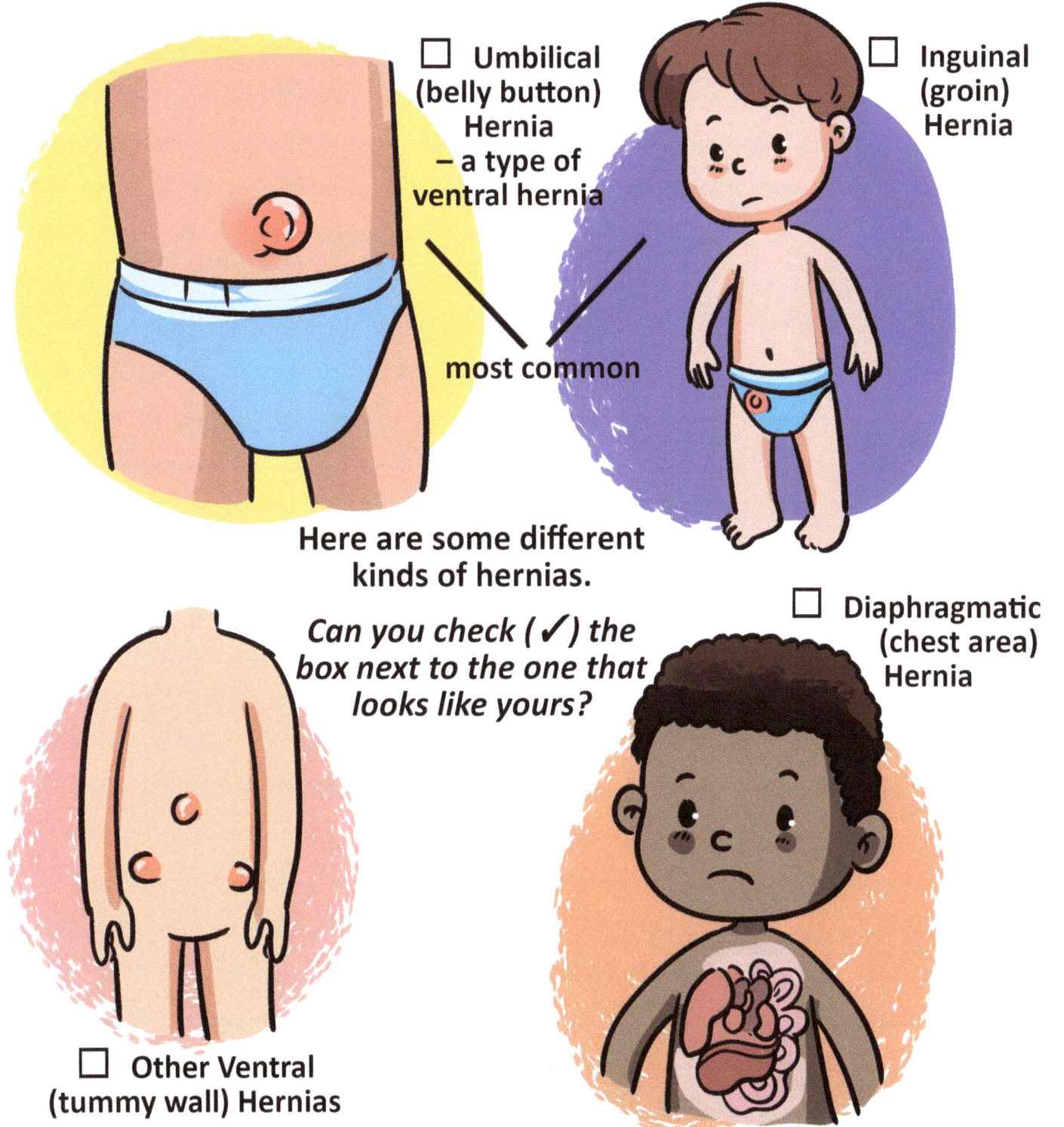

Don't worry! A hernia can be fixed with a surgery that makes the thin spot stronger.

Before surgery, you may meet your anesthesia and surgery doctors. They will check your hernia and tell you how you can help get ready.

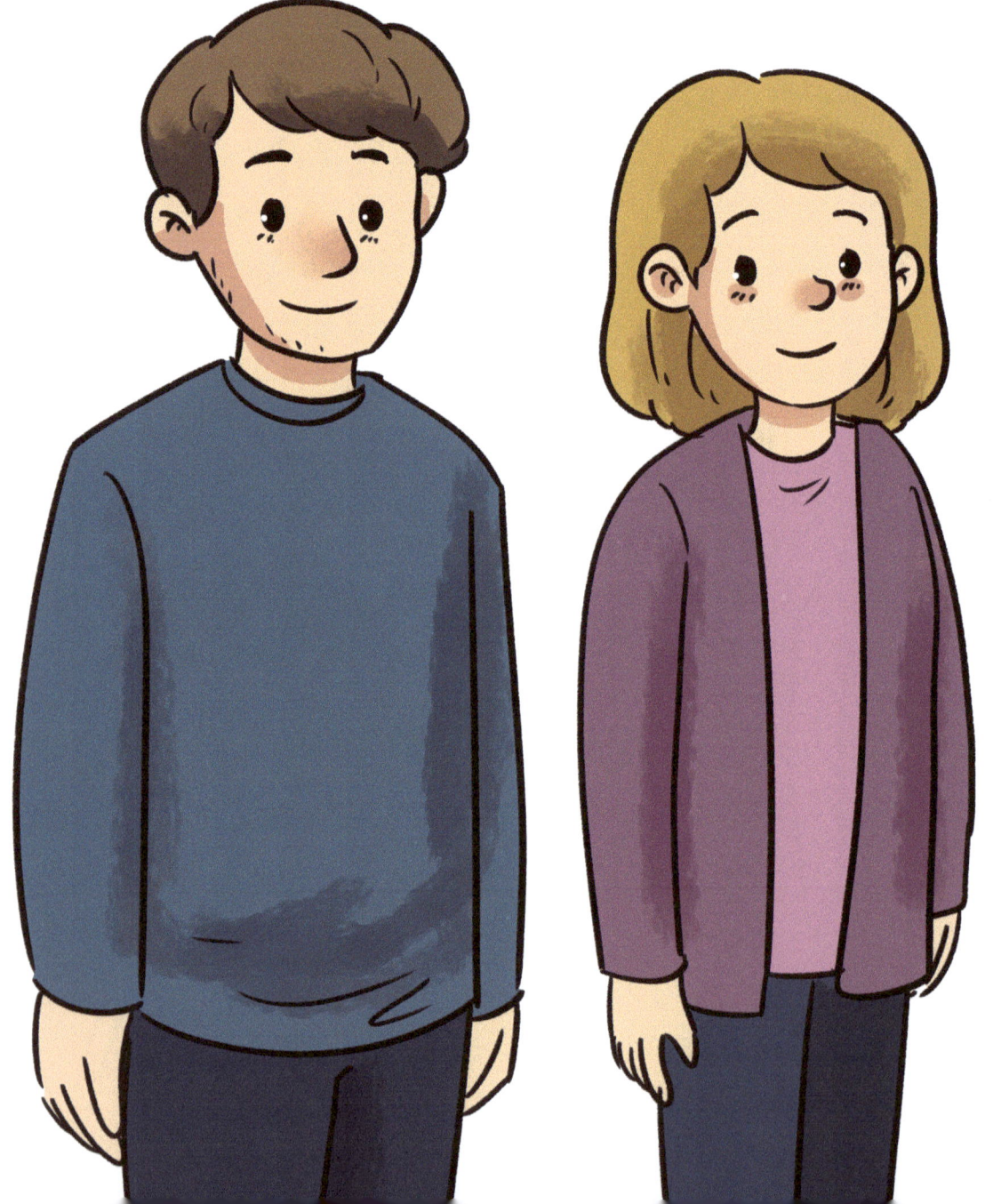

What kind of hernia do you have?
Put a checkmark (✓) in the box that matches yours!

☐ Inguinal   ☐ Umbilical   ☐ Other Ventral   ☐ Diaphragmatic

Where is your hernia?
Circle your answer:

Left   Right

   Middle

One of the most common hernias in children is an umbilical hernia. Most heal on their own by age 4 or 5, but if they don't, a doctor can fix it with a quick surgery.

While most hernias don't hurt, tell your parent or guardian right away if your hernia:

- feels sore or painful
- looks red or swollen
- feels hard

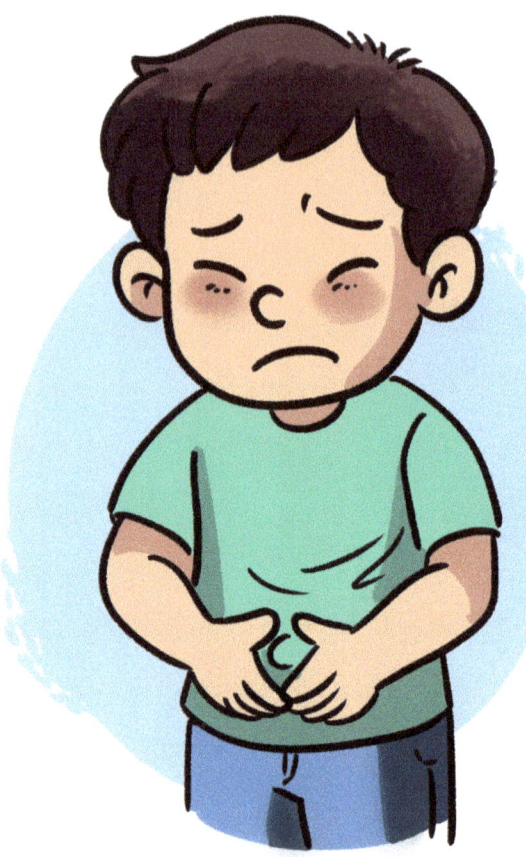

feels sore or painful

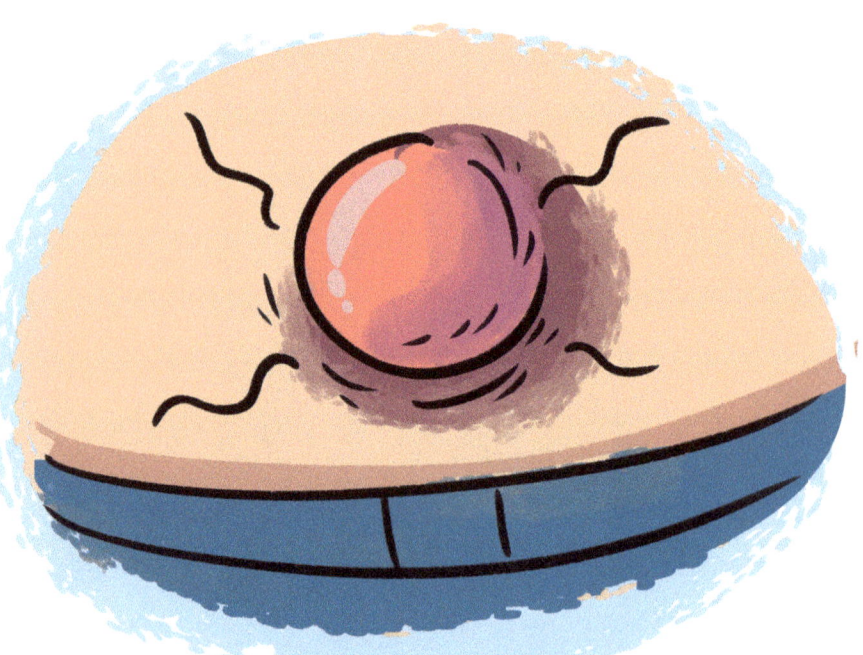

looks red or swollen

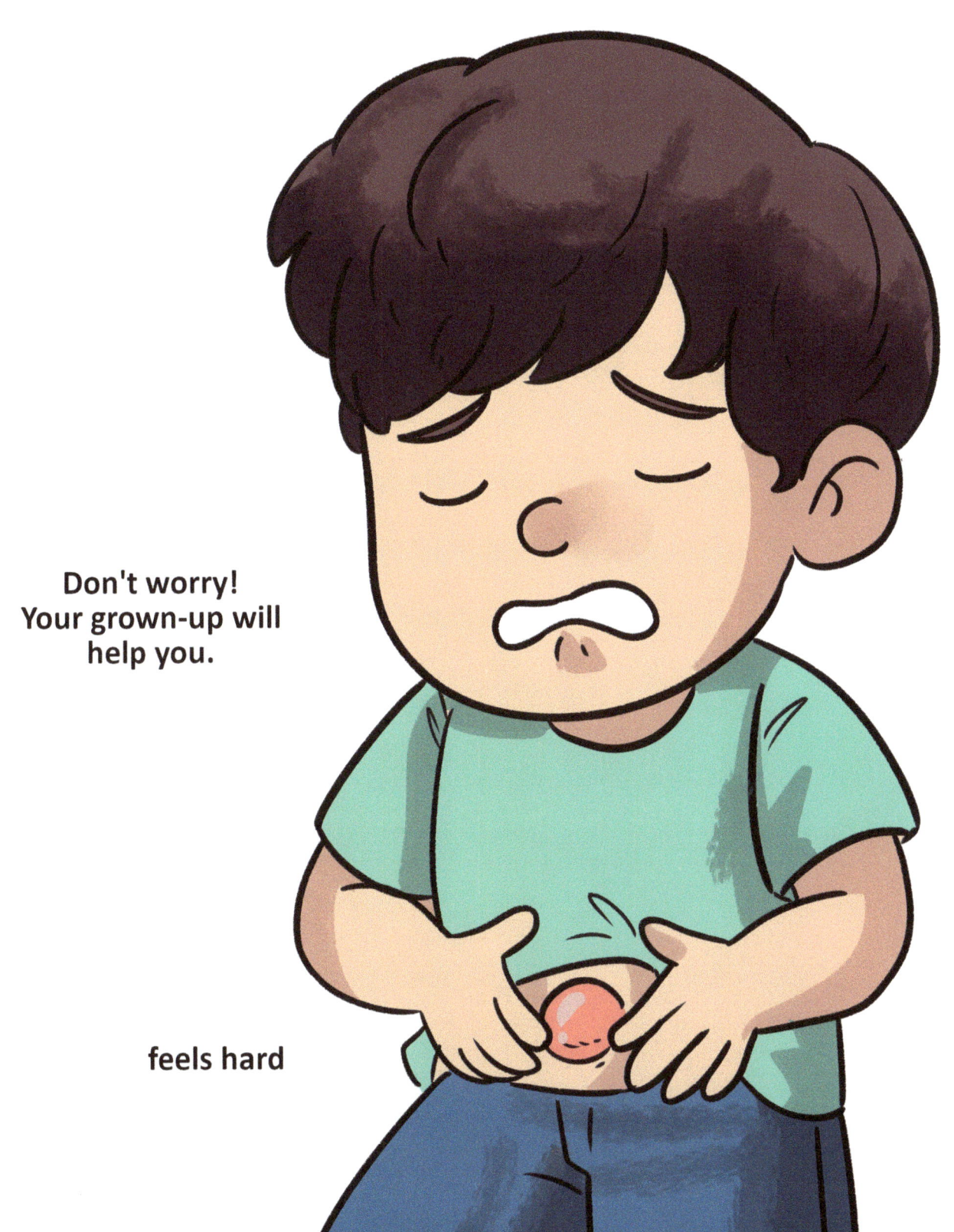

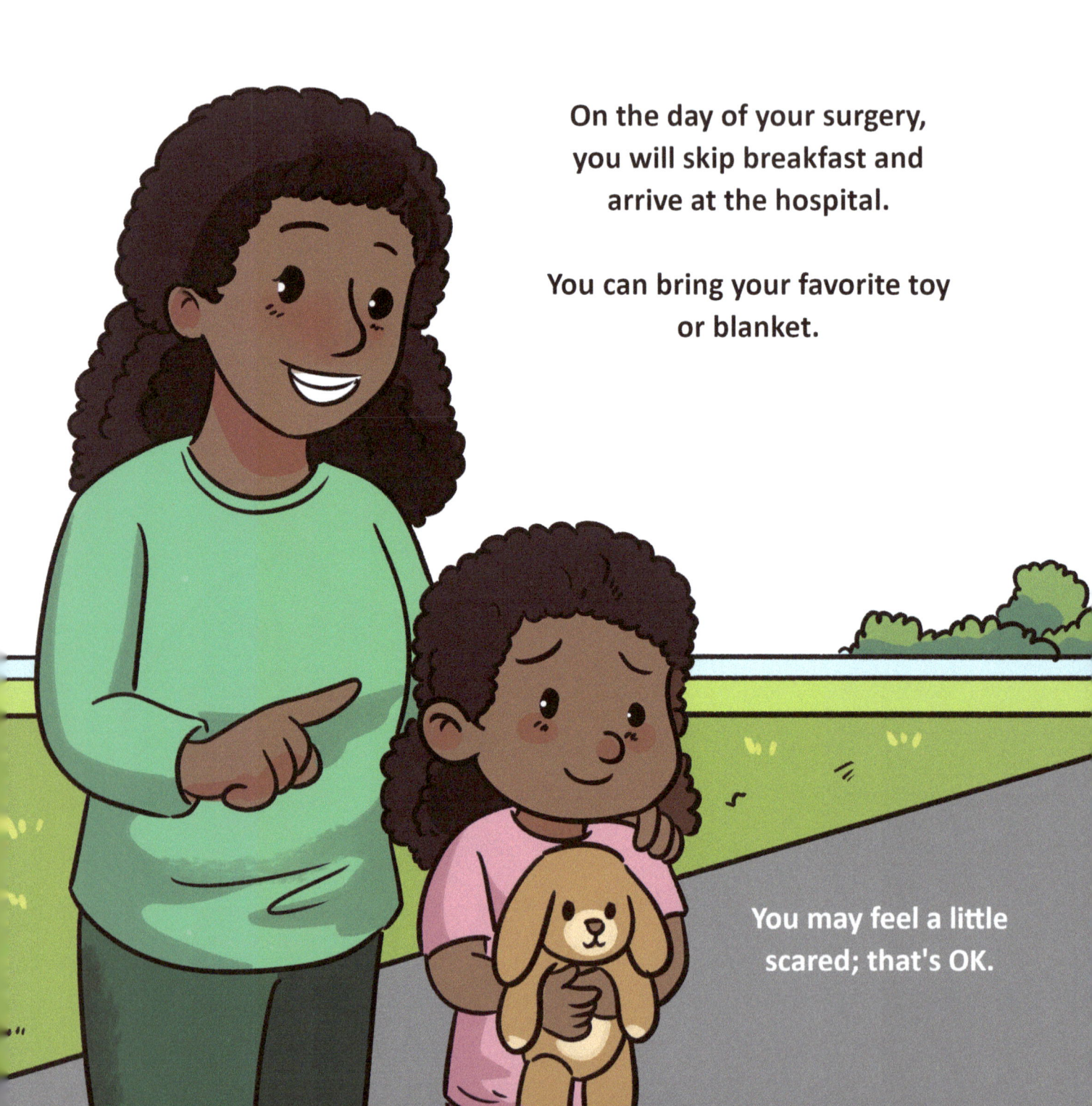

On the day of your surgery, you will skip breakfast and arrive at the hospital.

You can bring your favorite toy or blanket.

You may feel a little scared; that's OK.

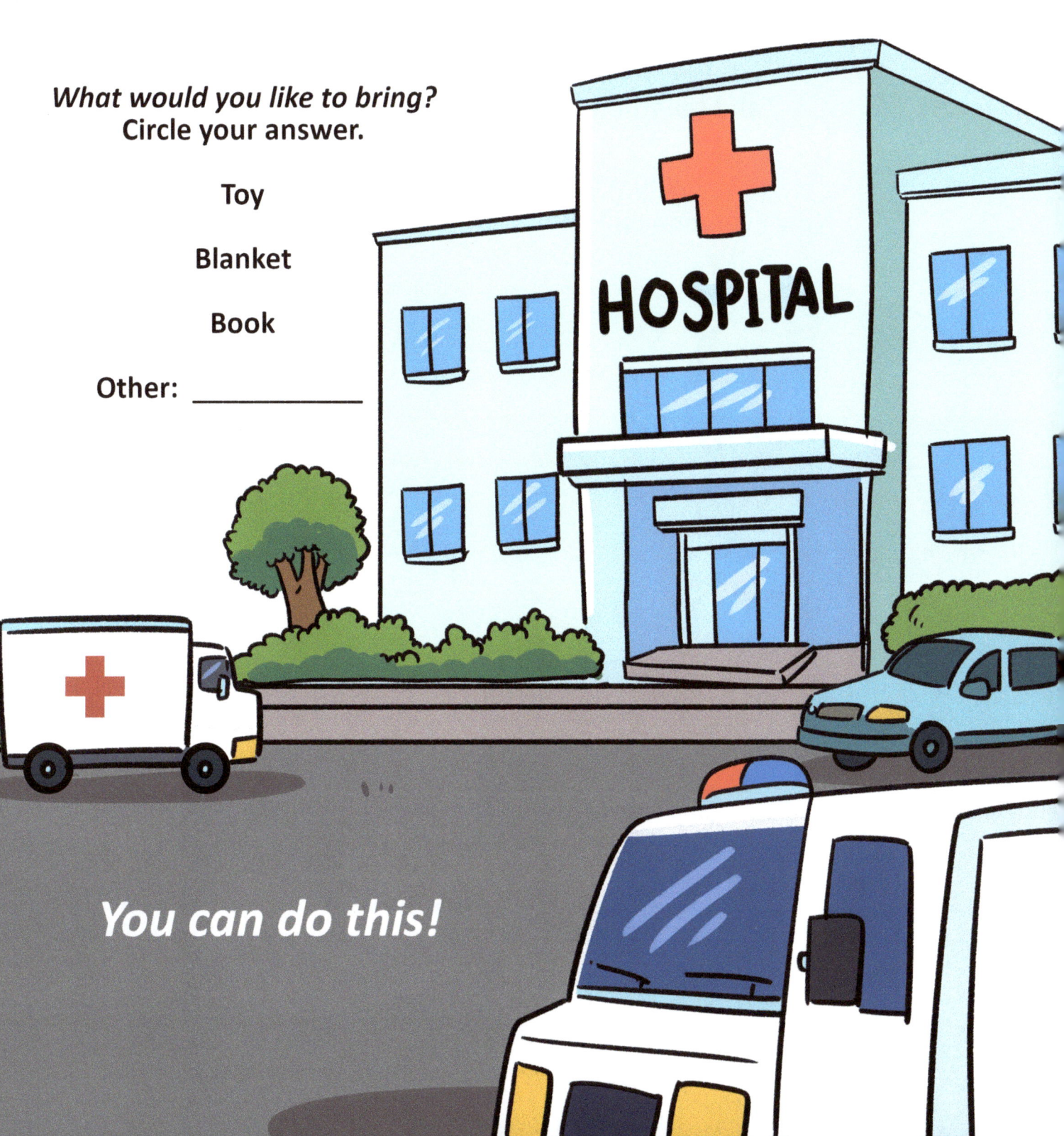

What would you like to bring?
Circle your answer.

Toy

Blanket

Book

Other: _____

You can do this!

You will check in at the hospital
and tell them your name and birthday.

Then, you will get a special wristband.
Now everyone will know your name and birthday!

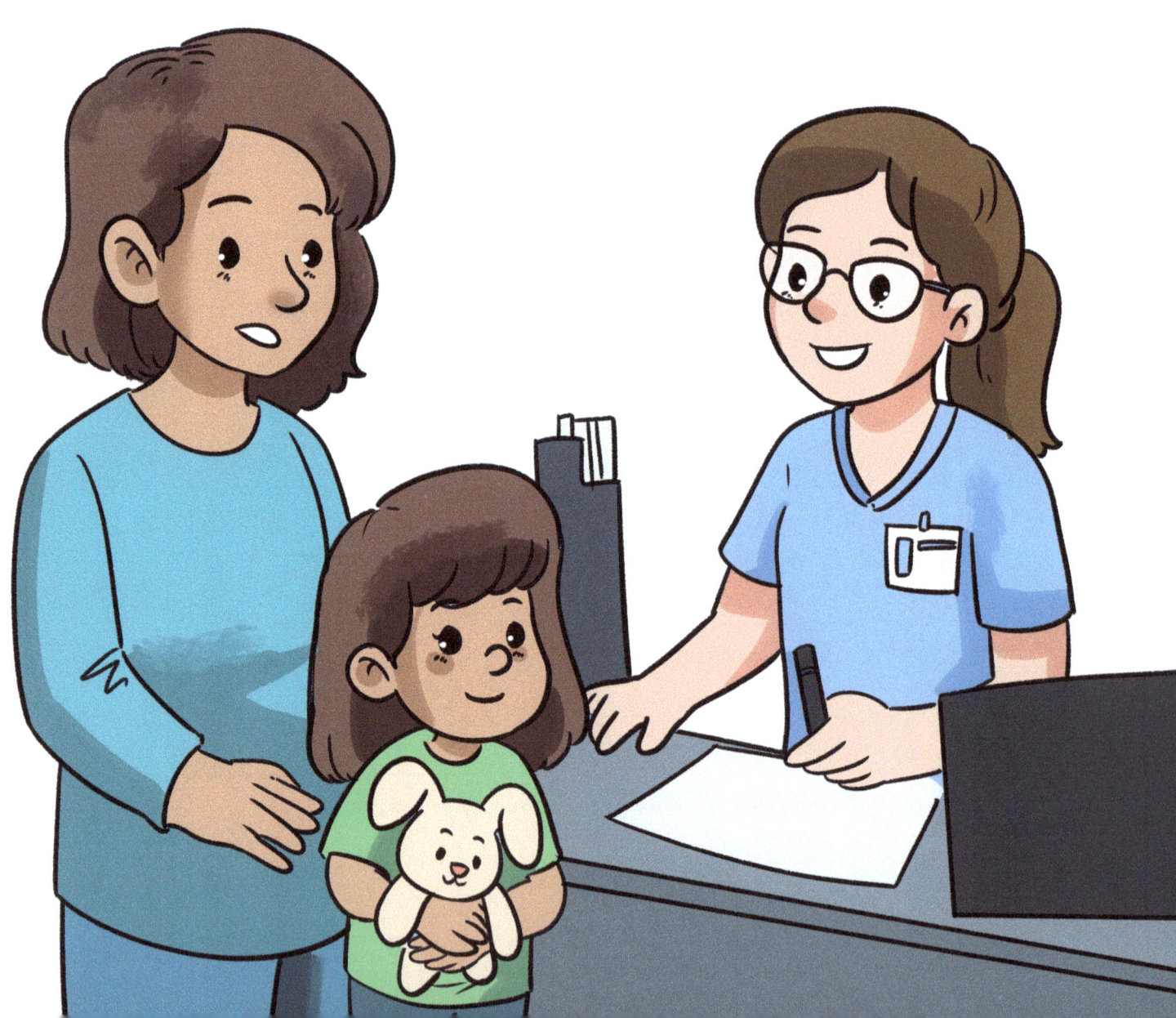

What color wristband will you get?
Circle the color of your wristband below.

Red　　Green　　Yellow　　Blue　　Pink　　Orange

Purple　　Black　　White

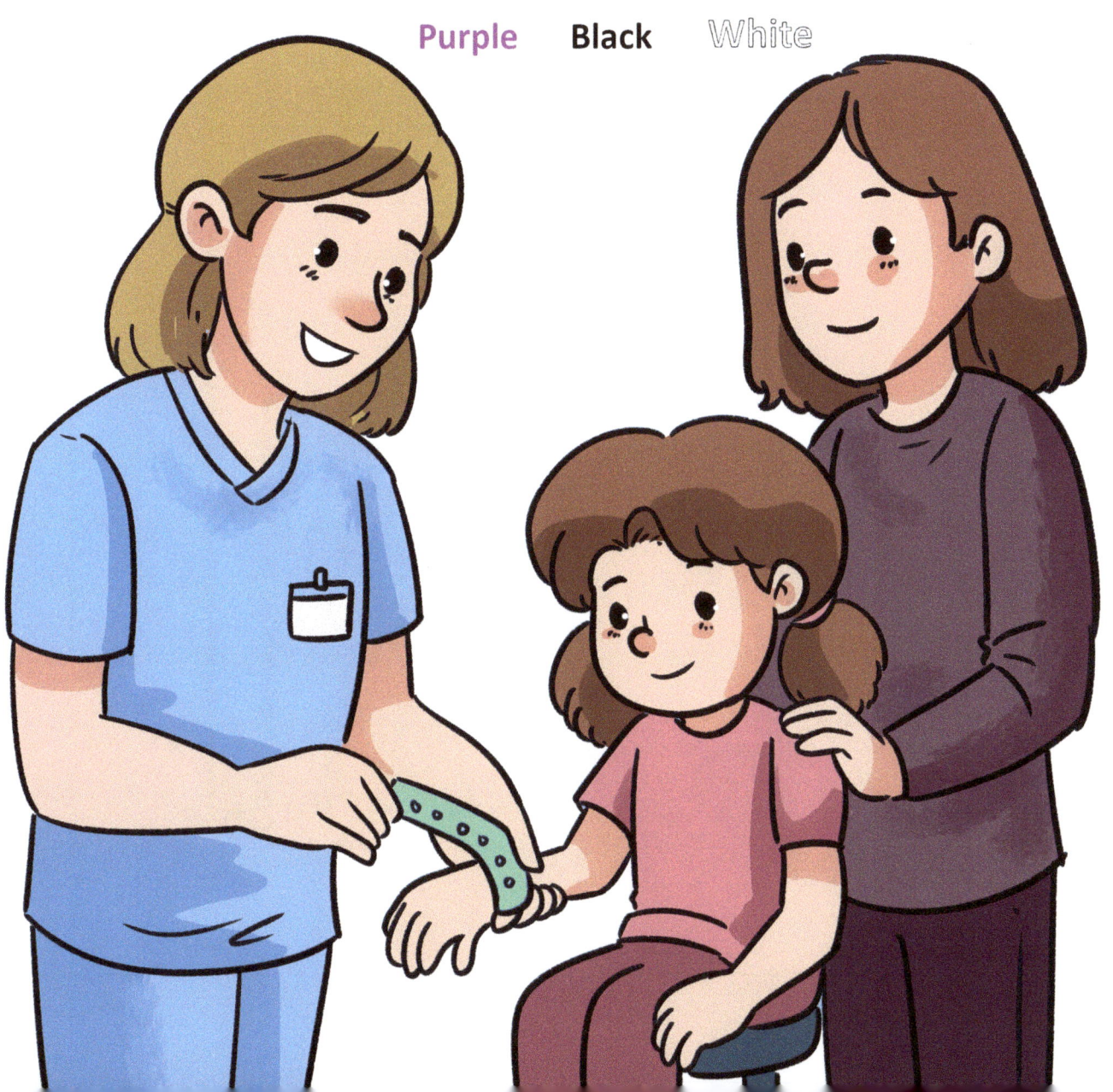

They will check your weight and height before getting you ready.

Do you know how much you weigh?

Do you know how tall you are?

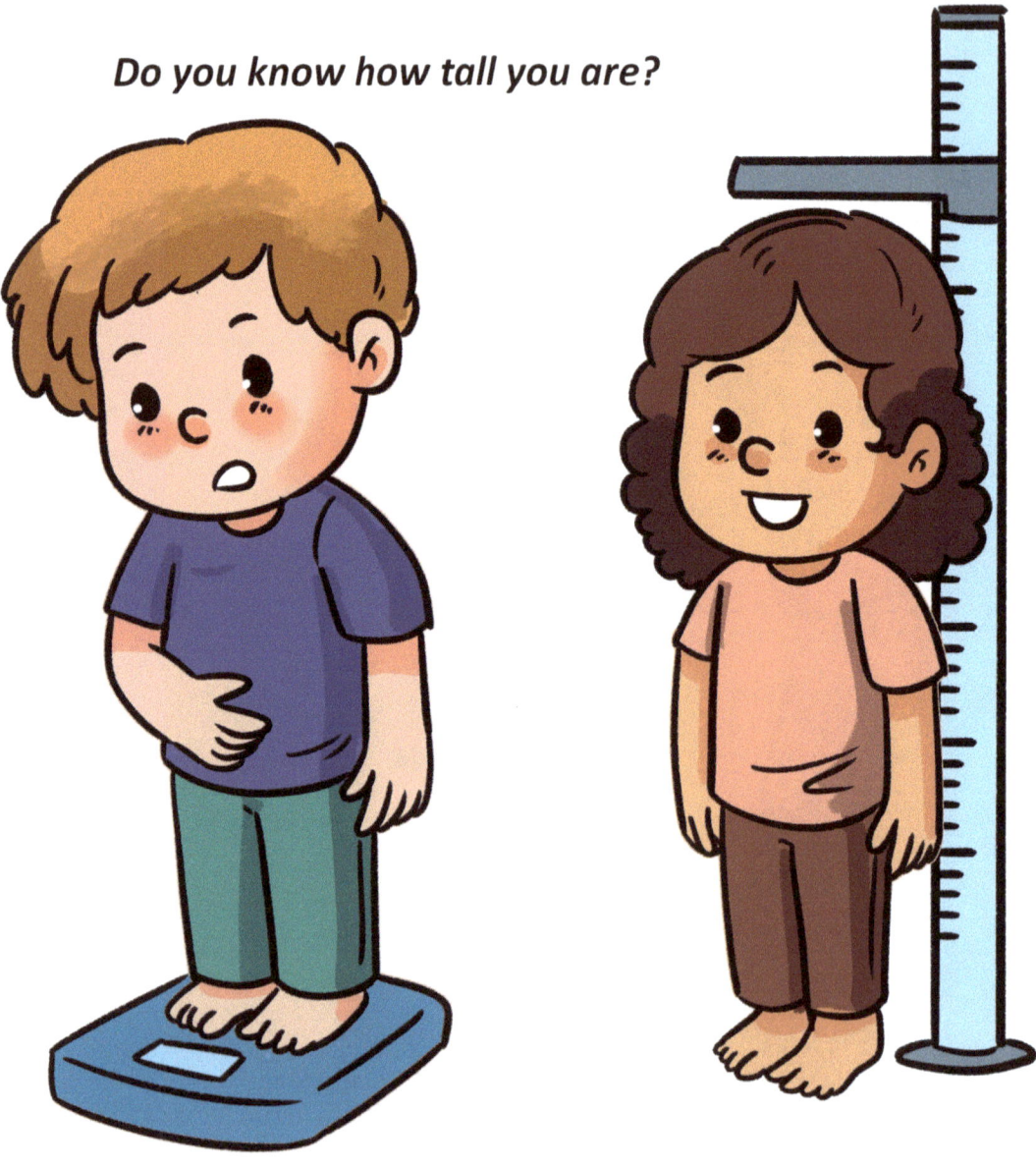

My weight is: _____   **My height is: _____**

You will change into a new outfit, put on a hat, a gown (that looks like a backward superhero cape), and some cozy socks.

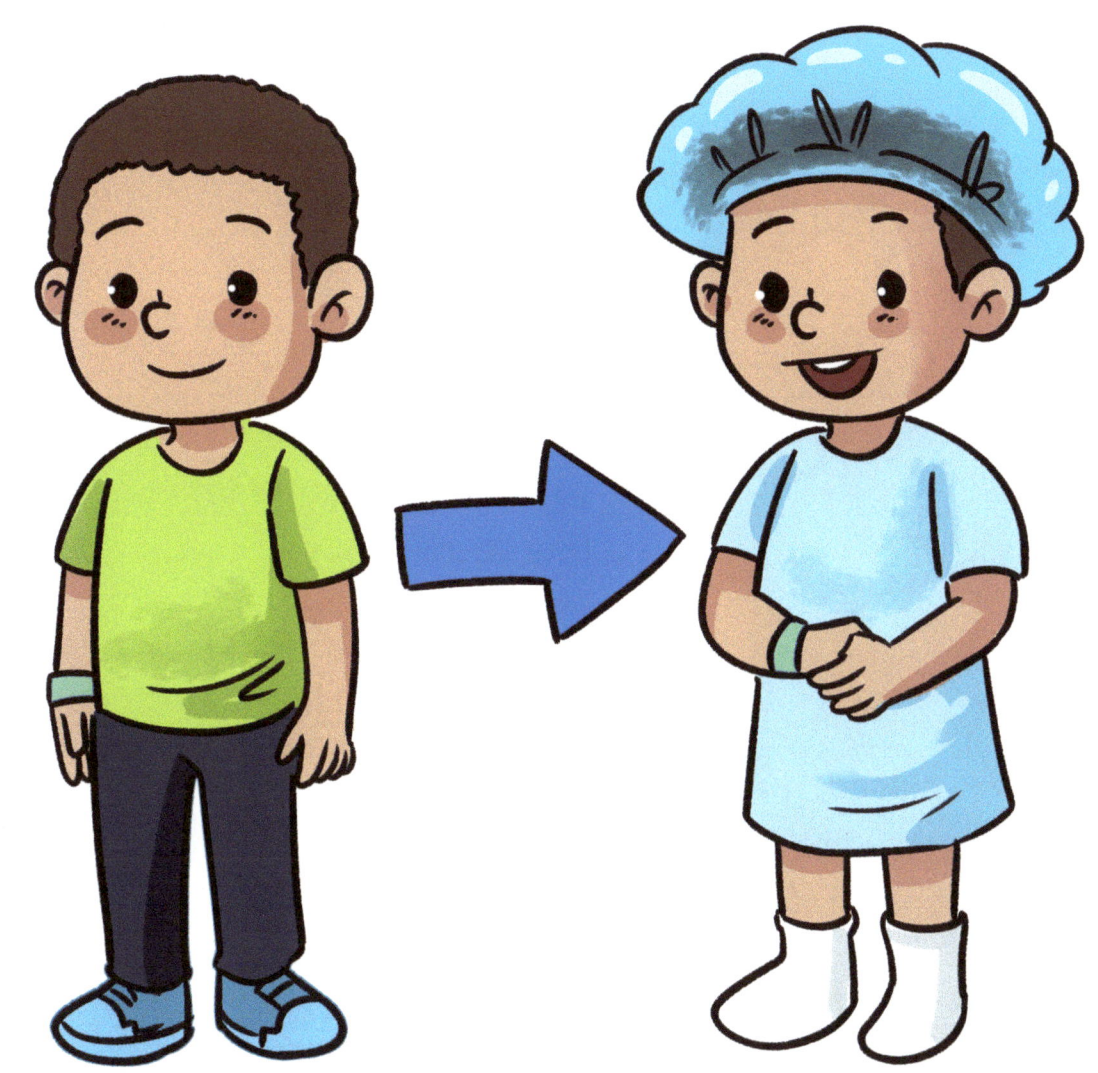

You've got this!

Your nurse may use a clip to check how much oxygen is in your body.

Which finger or toe do you want to use?

Oxygen helps your body work,
so you can do all the things you love!

What do you love to do?

You will need an IV for your surgery.
It's a tiny straw that gives your body medicine.

Sometimes it is placed before you fall asleep.
It may feel like a quick poke.

Before it is placed, numbing cream can be used to help your skin feel more comfortable.

Other times, the IV is placed after you are asleep.

Your doctors and nurses will choose the safest way.

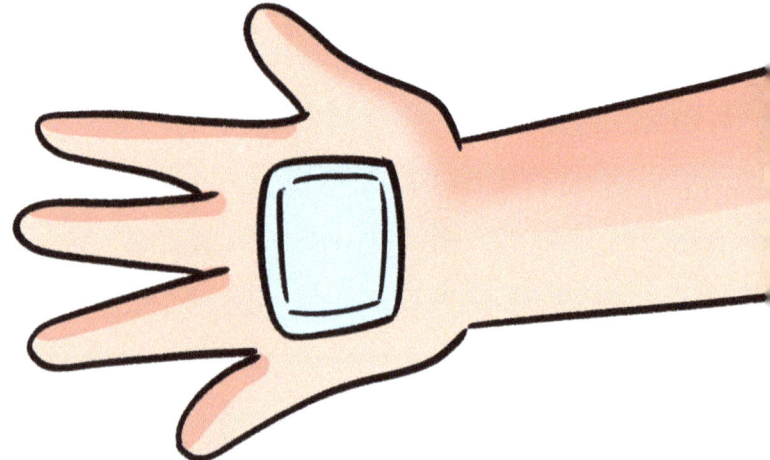

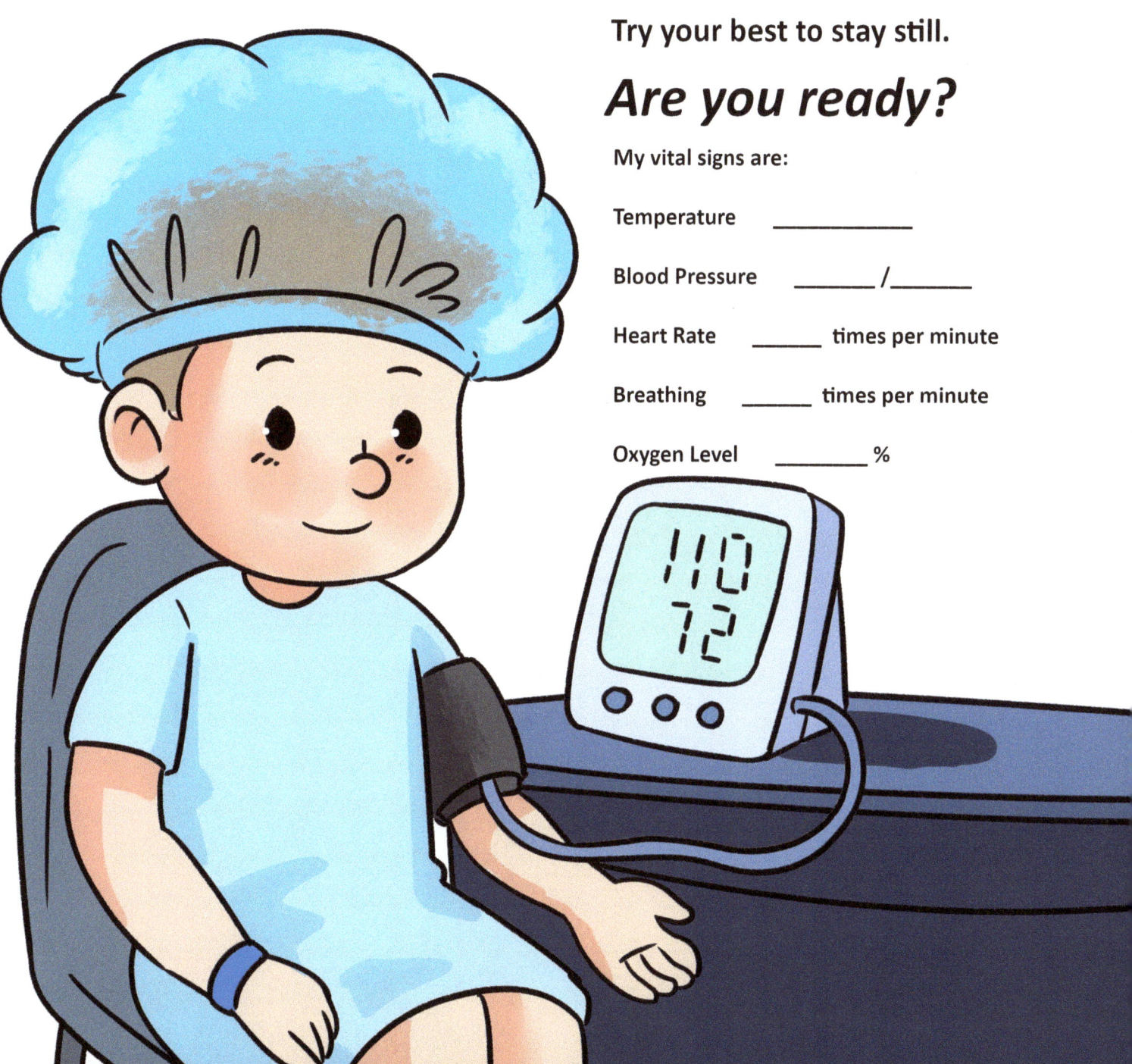

Before your surgery, you and your grown-up will meet the doctors and nurses who will take care of you.

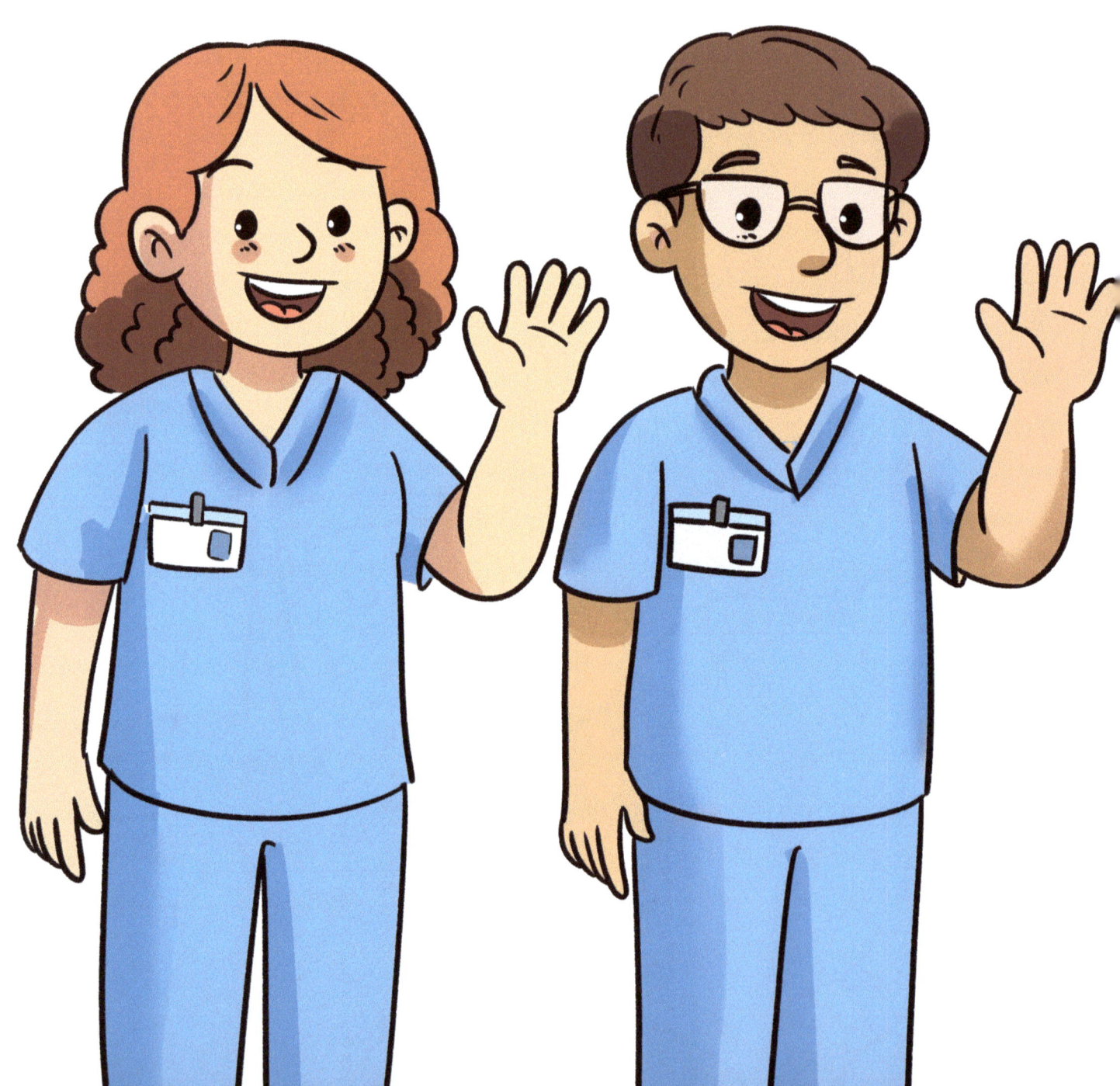

They are gentle and careful, and they'll help you feel better.
They're also happy to answer any questions you have.
If you have any questions, feel free to ask!

You may get a special, sweet medicine to help you feel more calm.

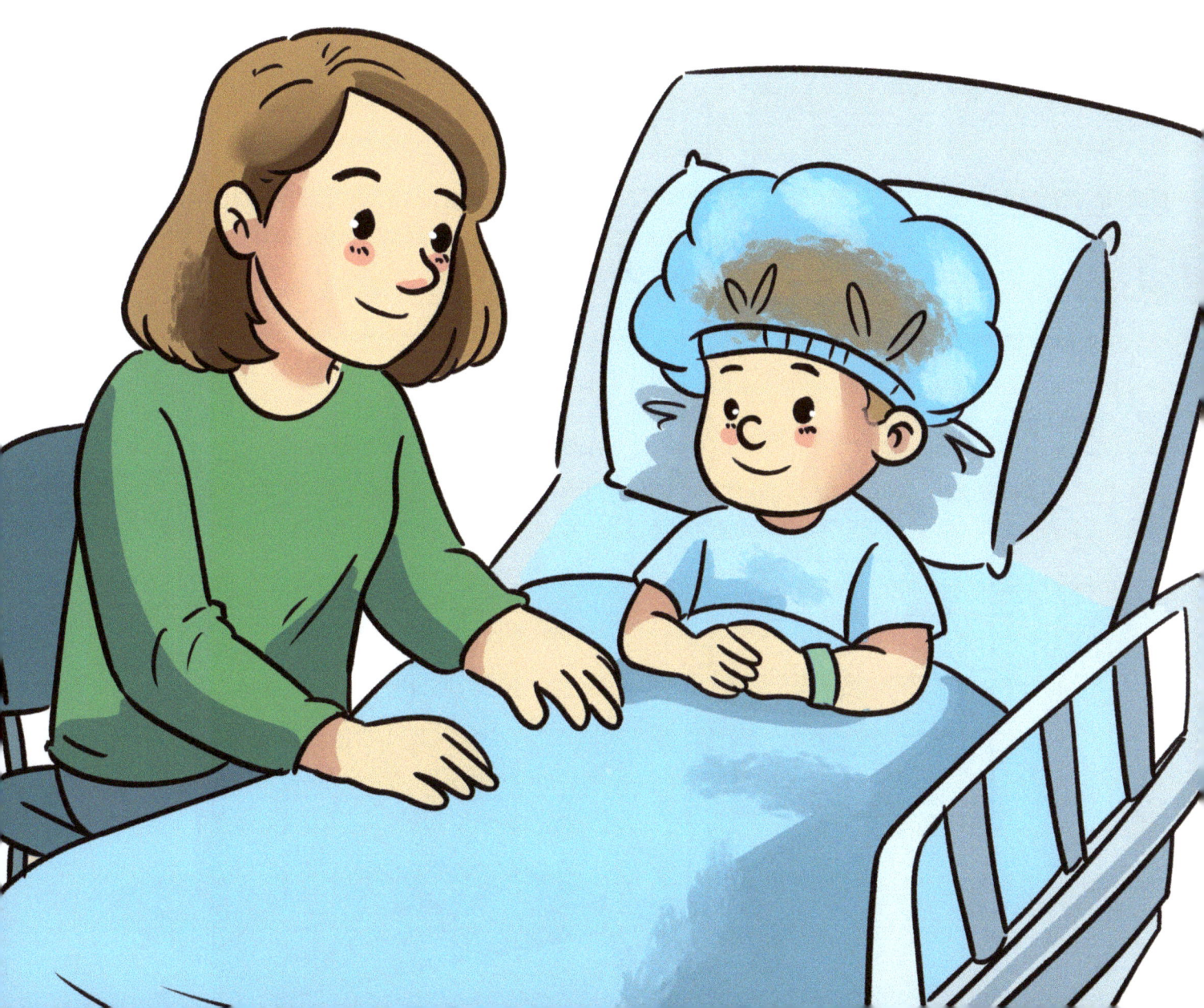

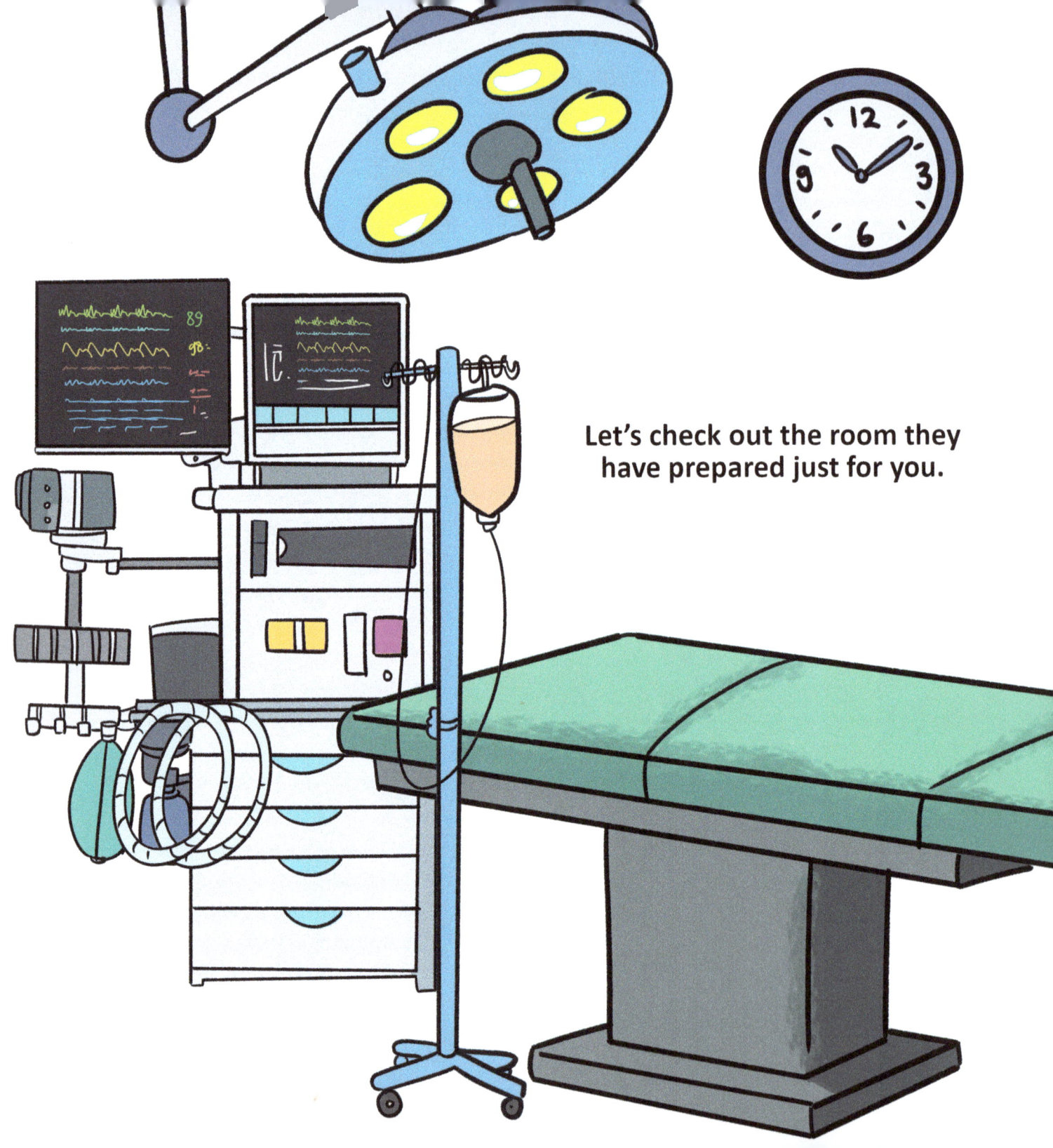

Can you find these things in the room?

- ☐ Bright lights hanging from the ceiling
- ☐ Surgery staff wearing masks
- ☐ An IV (intravenous) pole for hanging bags of fluids and medicine
- ☐ An anesthesia machine with a balloon attached to it
- ☐ A clock
- ☐ A warm bed just for you

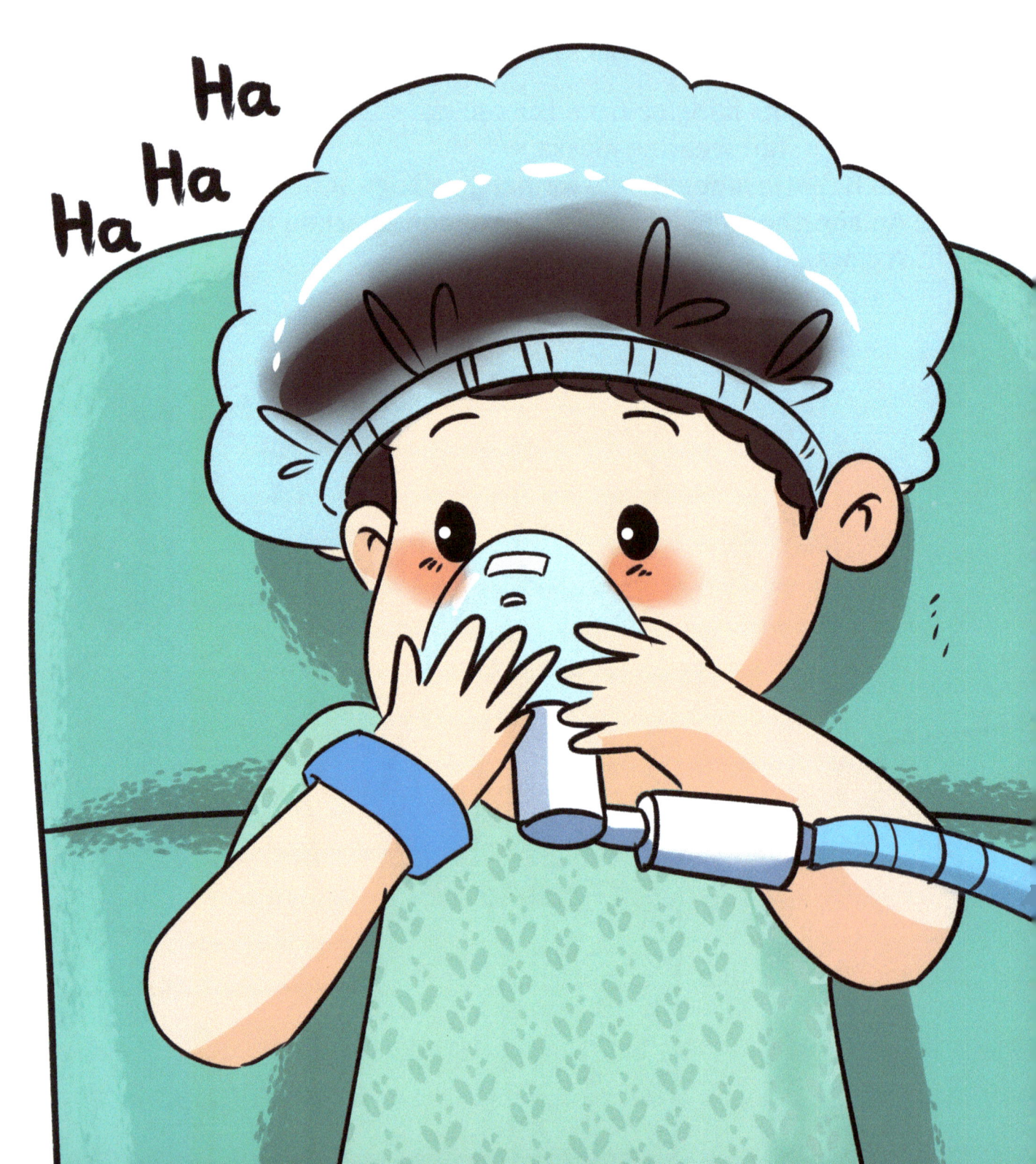

Once you're on the bed, your anesthesia doctor will give you laughing gas through a mask to help you fall asleep.

Did you know they can make your mask smell sweet and yummy like bubble gum or your favorite fruit?

Draw or write down what scent you would like your mask to smell like:

_____

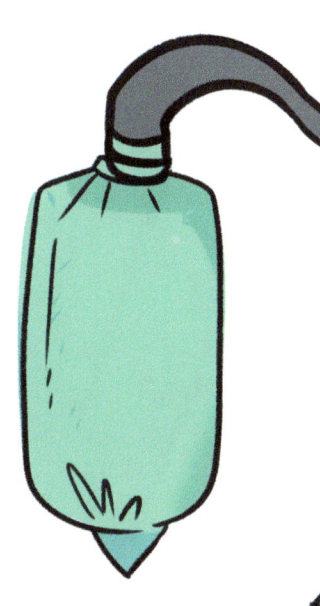

You can also watch your breathing by looking at the balloon on the anesthesia machine.

Cool, right?

<u>Challenge</u>: Can you blow into your mask and make the balloon bigger?

If you already have an IV in your hand, the sleeping medicine will go through that instead.

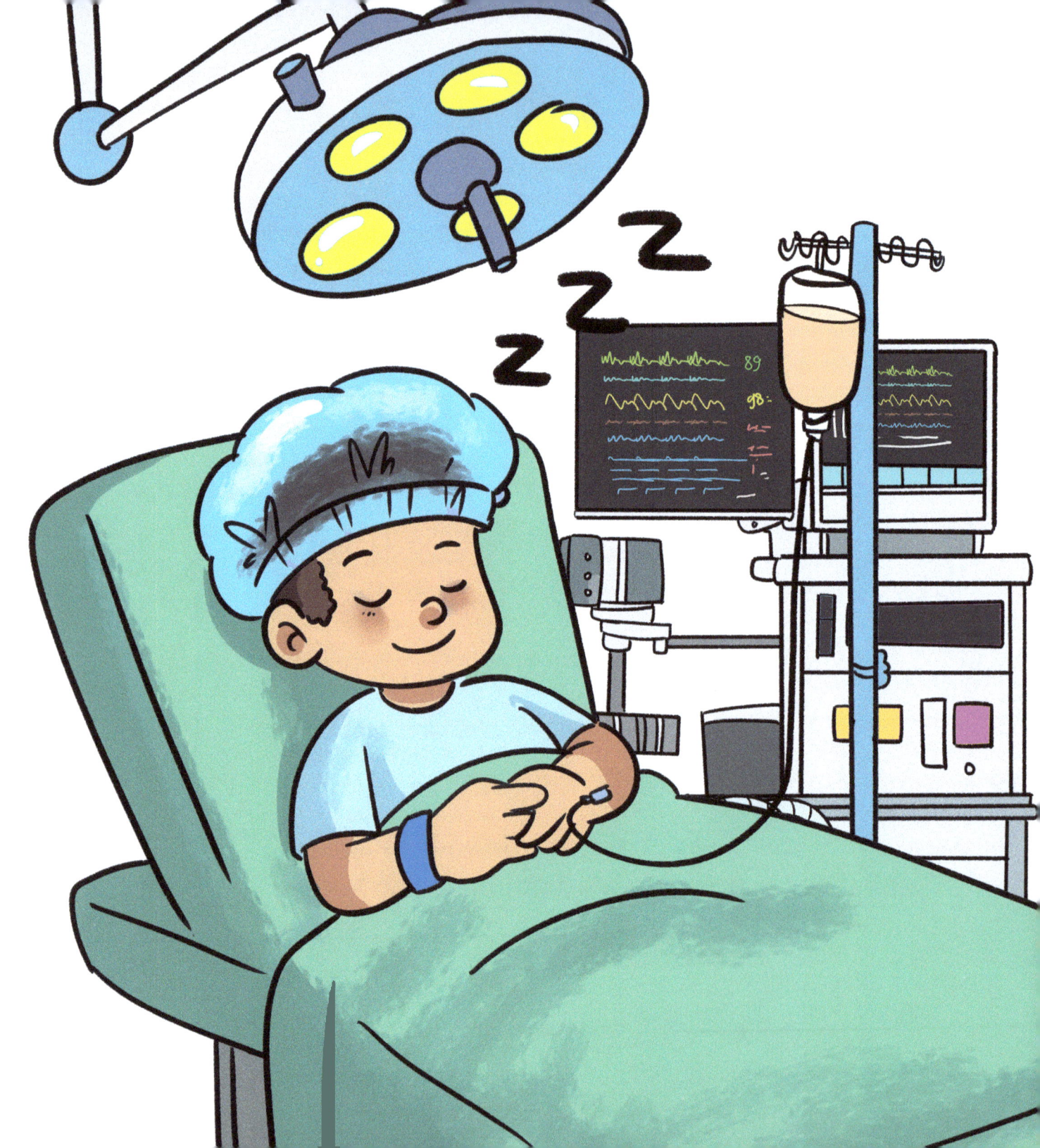

Soon, you will feel sleepy and want to take a nap.

Do you have a nice dream picked out?

What would you like to dream about?

During the surgery, your surgeon will gently and carefully fix your hernia.

Your surgery will be done while you're dreaming away, and you won't feel a thing!

Your nurses and doctors will take good care of you and keep you safe and comfortable.

Sweet dreams...

You're so brave!

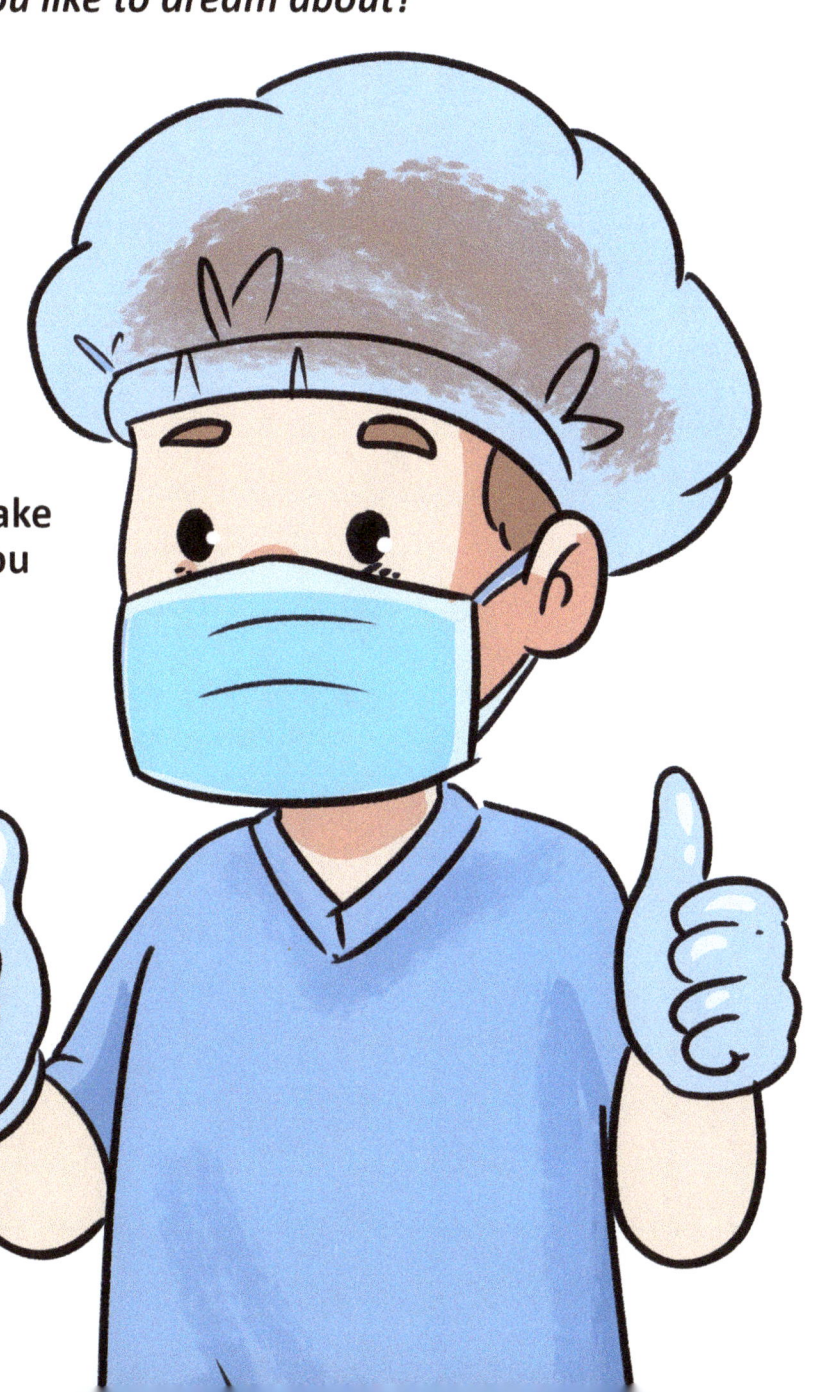

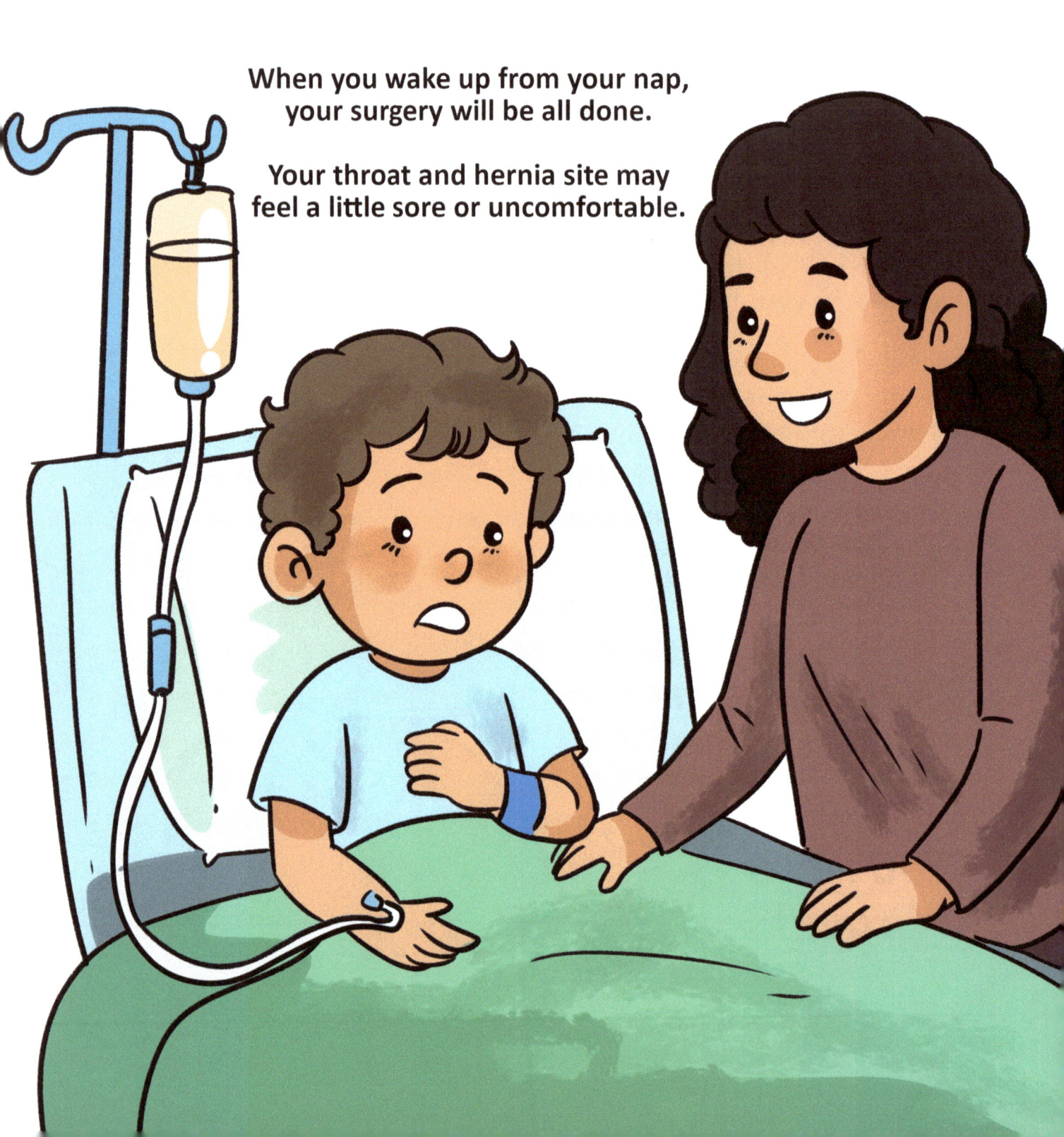

If you need medicine to help you feel better, it will be given to you through the small straw in your arm or leg.

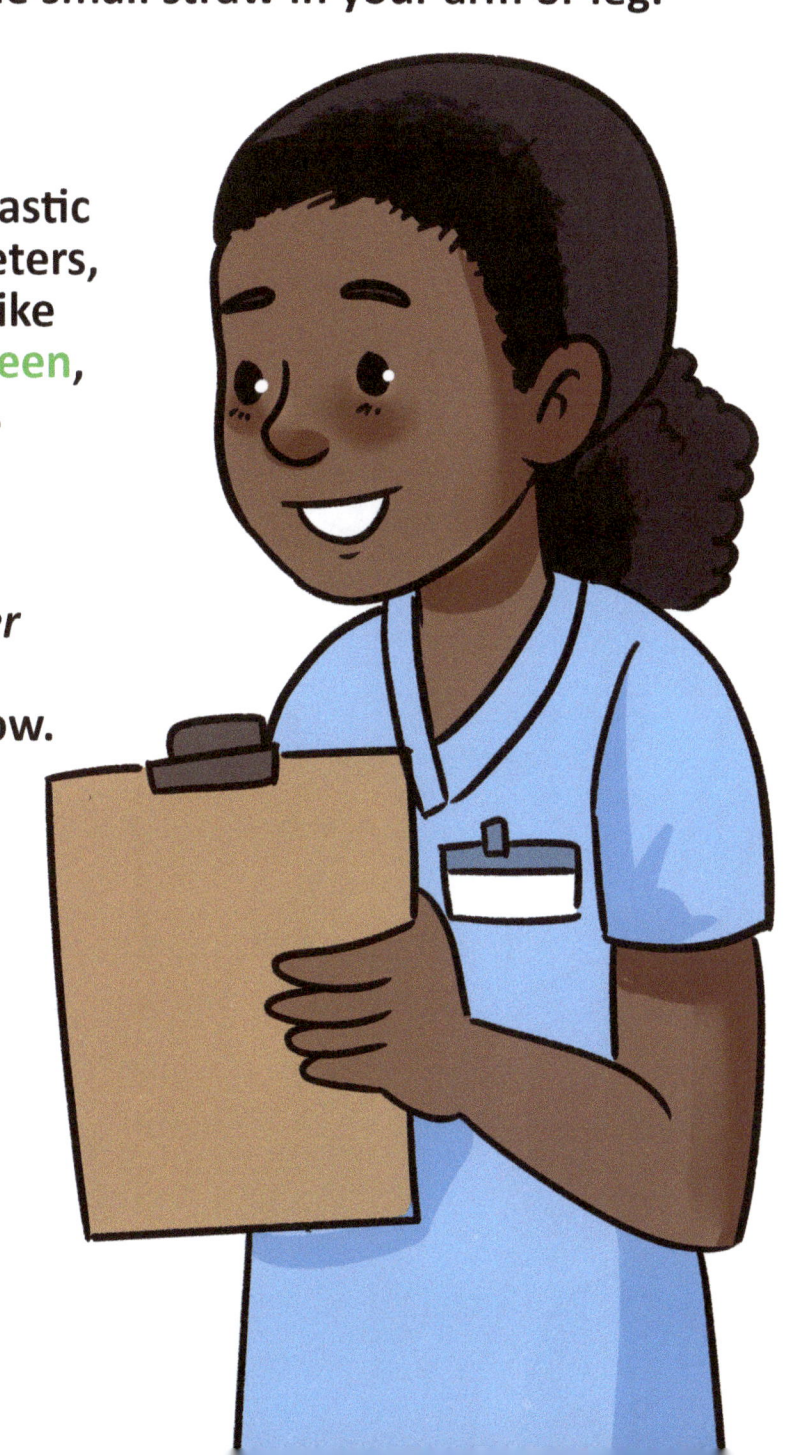

Fun fact: The small plastic straws, called IV catheters, come in fun colors like yellow, blue, pink, green, gray, and orange.

What color IV catheter will you get?
Circle your IV color below.

yellow   blue

pink   green

gray   orange

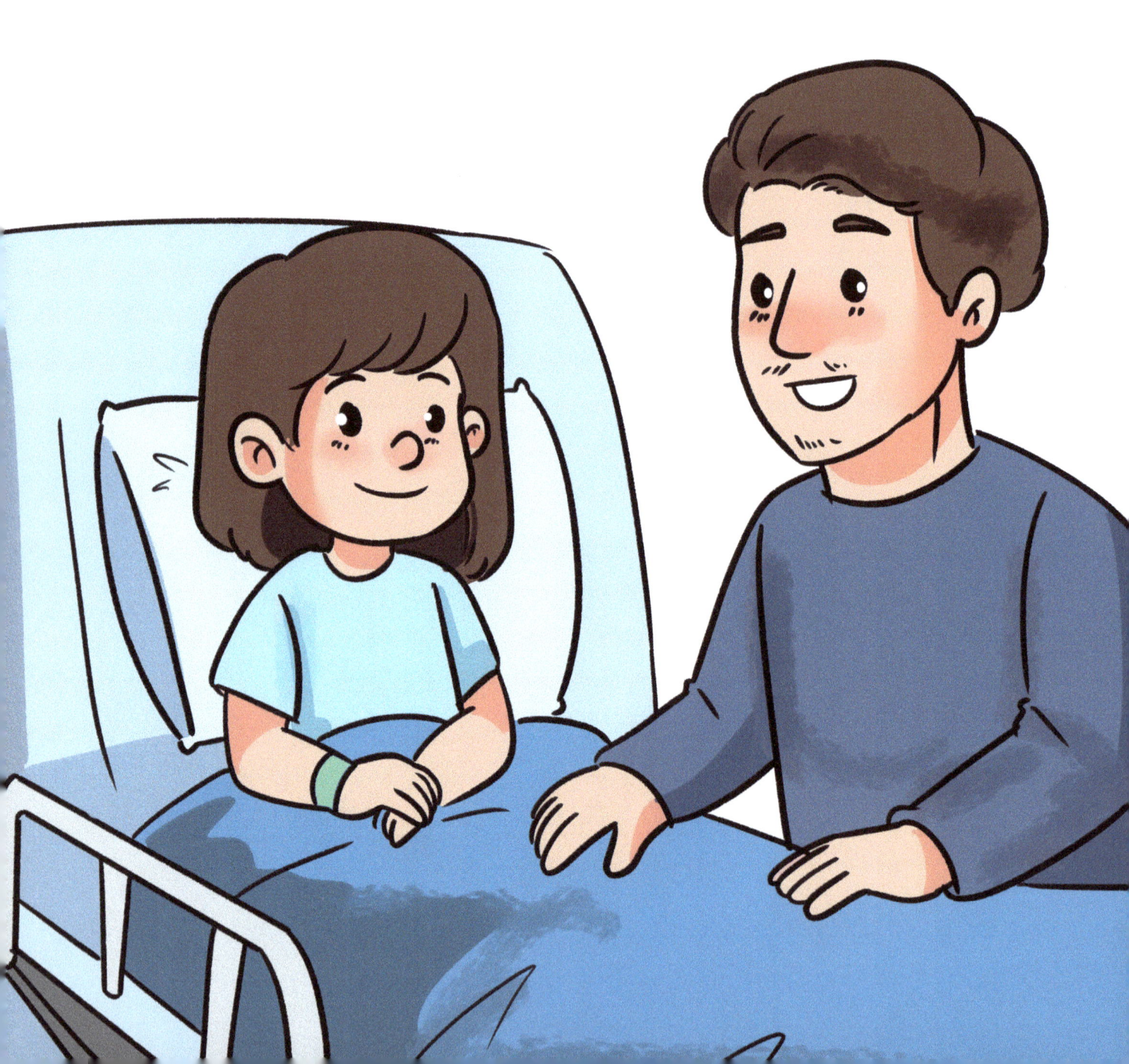

Usually, you can go home the same day.

If you need to stay in the hospital, your parent or guardian can stay with you to help you feel safe and comfortable.

You'll go home when you're feeling better and stronger.

What are some things that will help you feel better and more comfortable after your hernia surgery?
Put a checkmark next to your favorites!

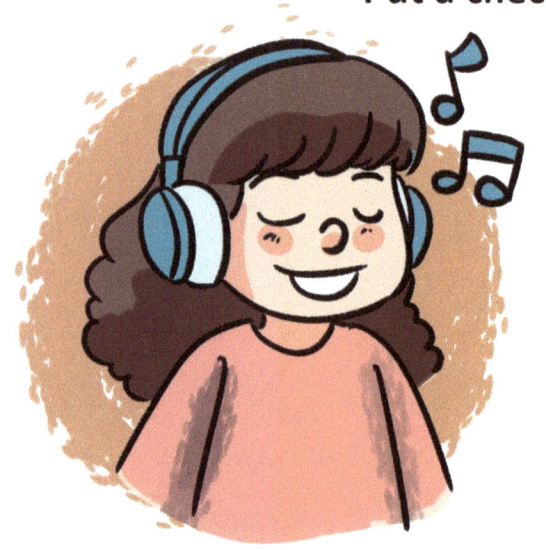

☐ listen to music and sing along

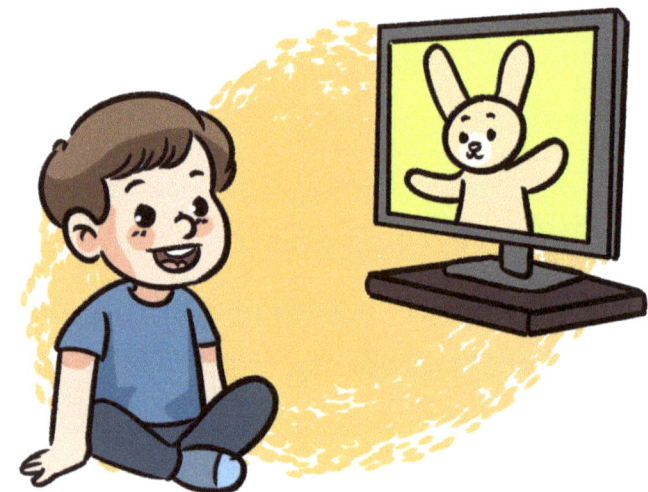

☐ watch your favorite show

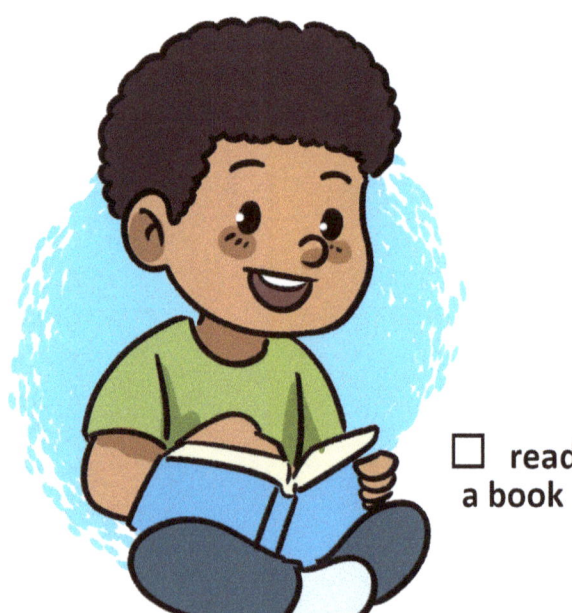

☐ read a book

☐ get a gentle massage

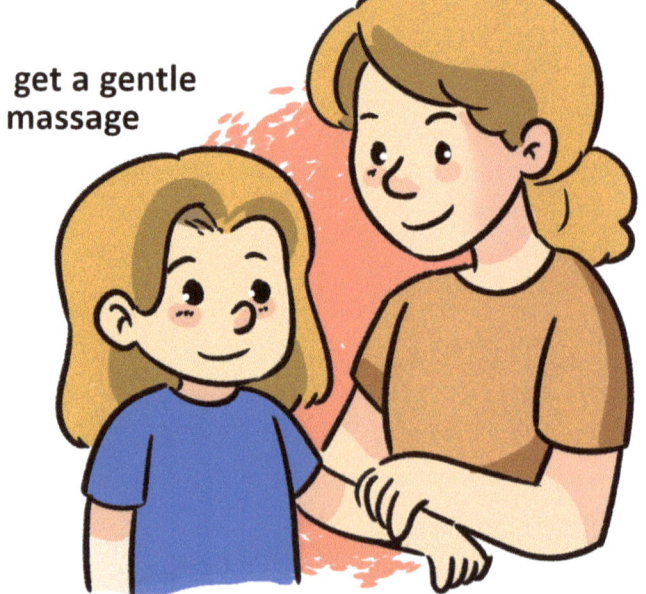

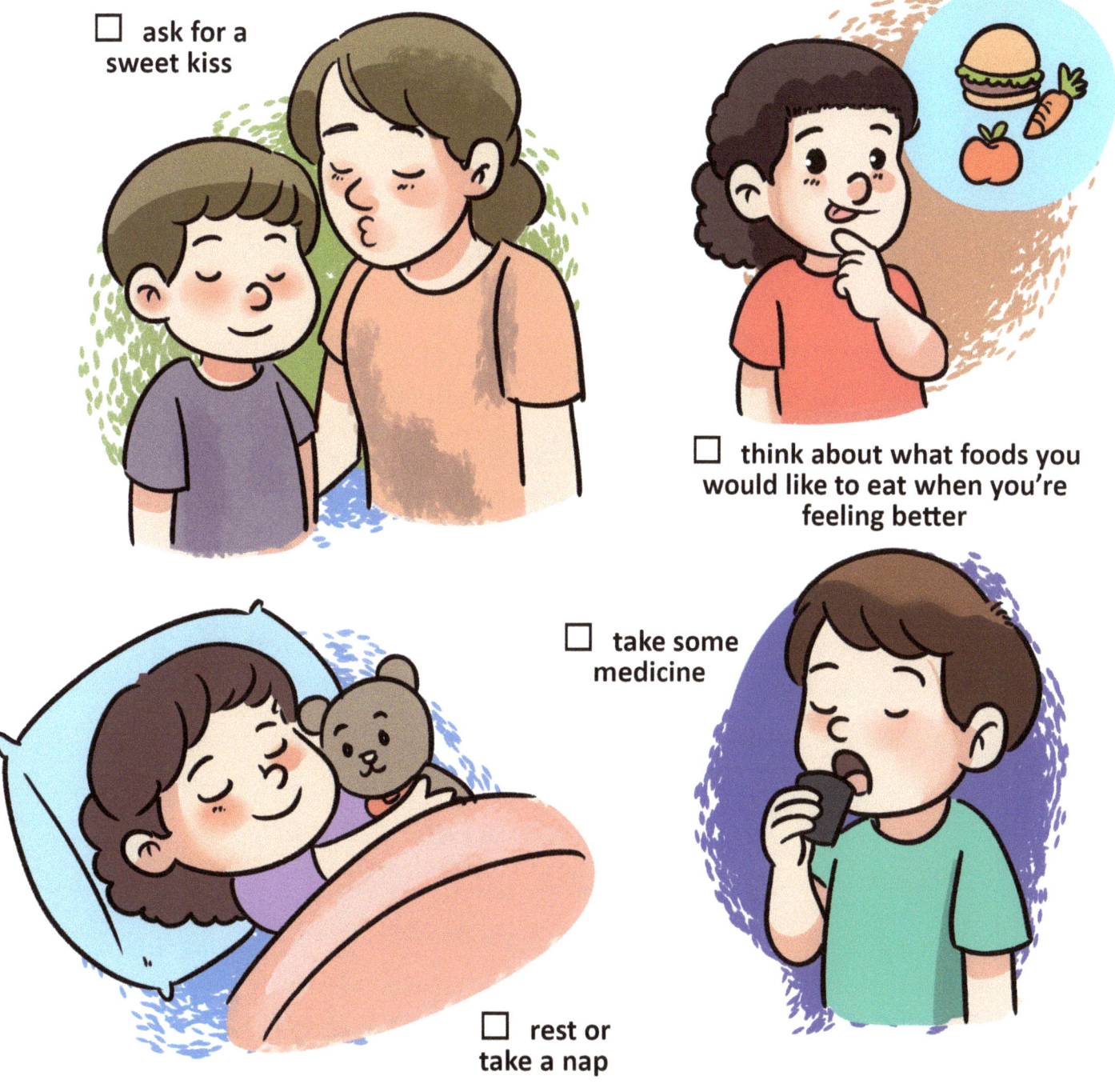

After your surgery, you won't be able to do some activities until your scar has had time to heal.

Don't worry! Your doctor will tell your parent or guardian how to help you and when it's safe to do these activities again.

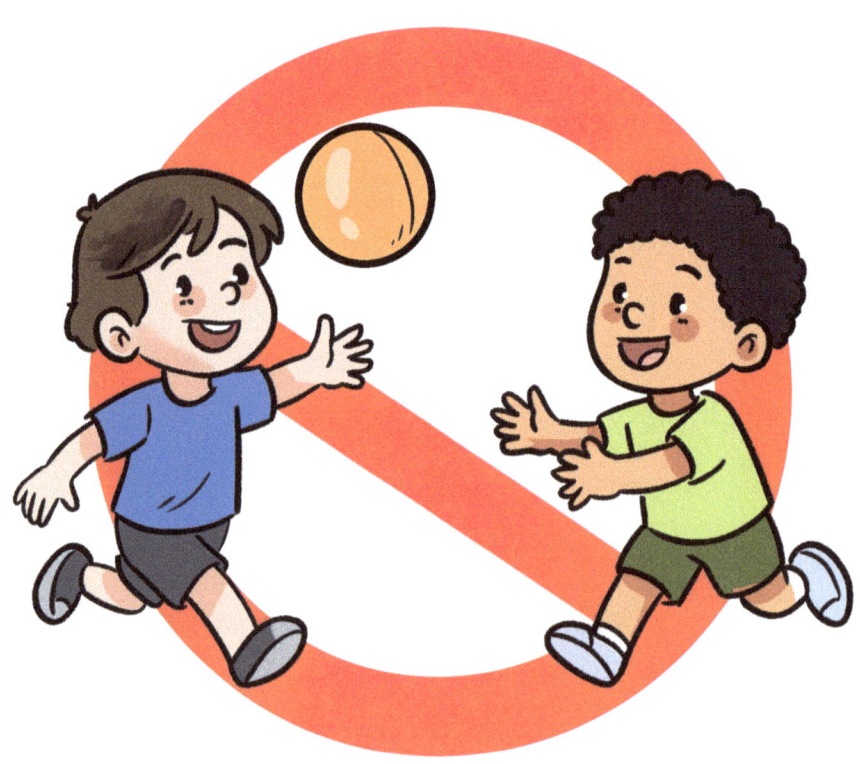

No contact sports (where players can bump into each other)

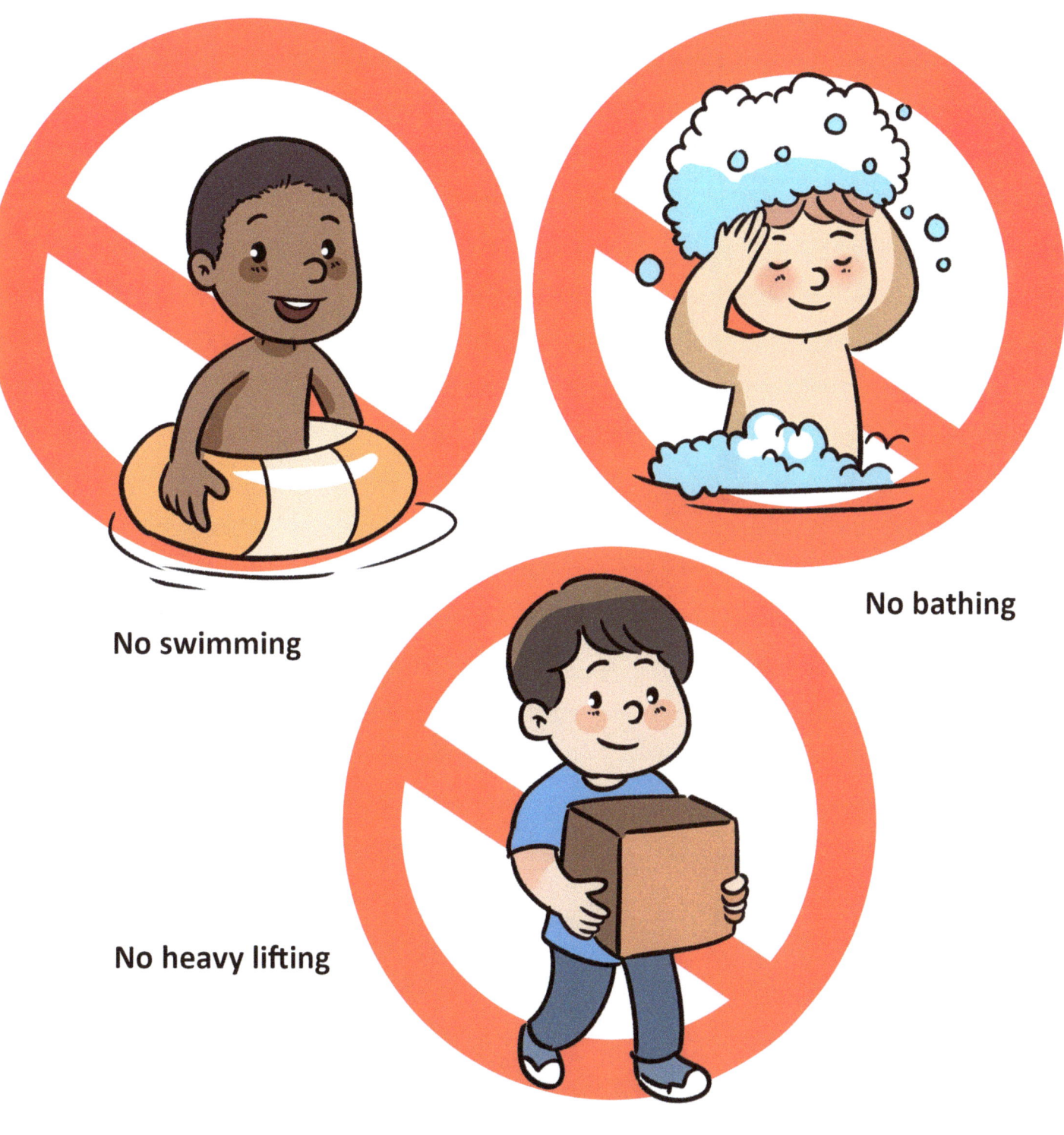

When you're feeling better, eat healthy foods and stay hydrated.

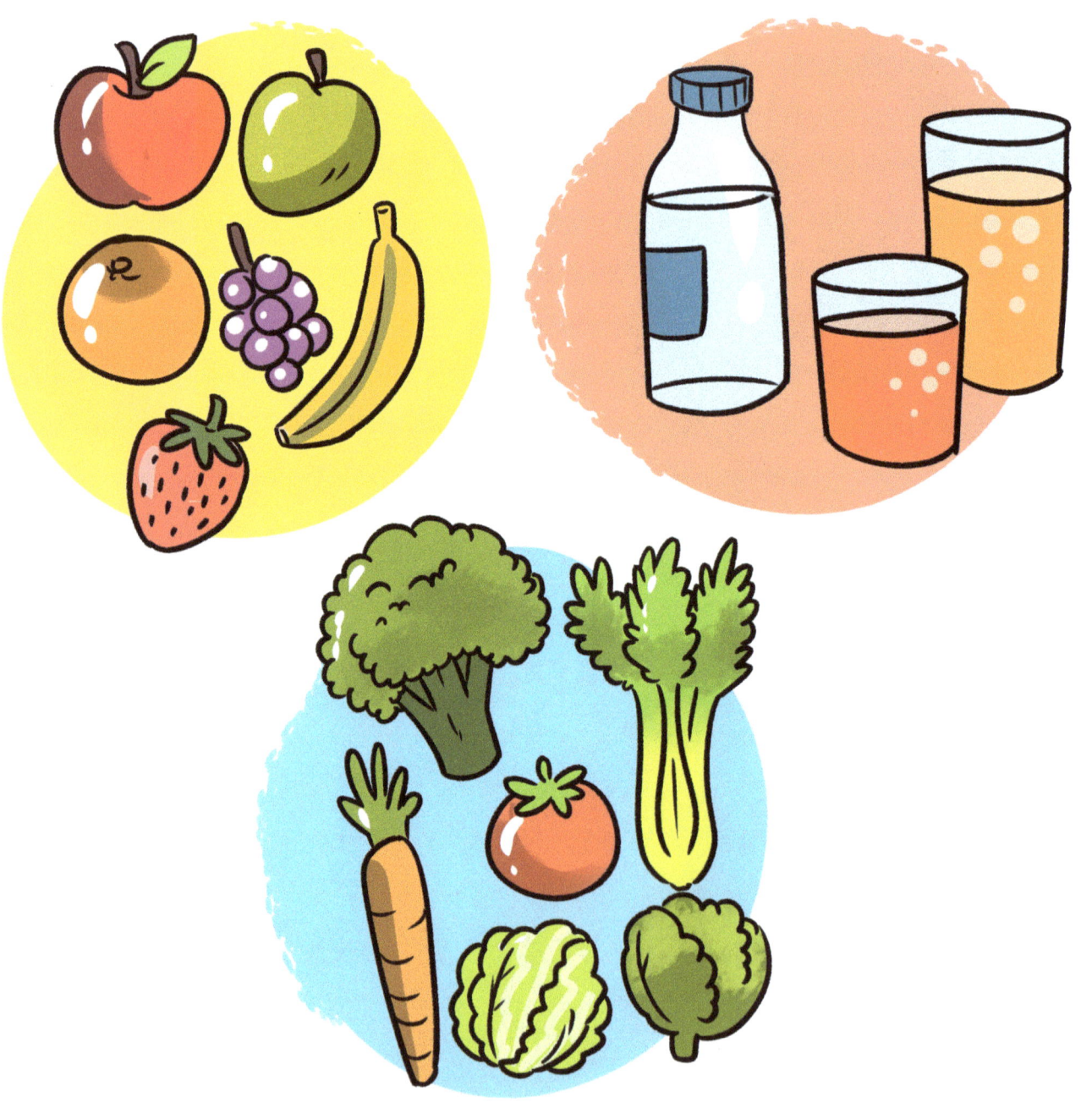

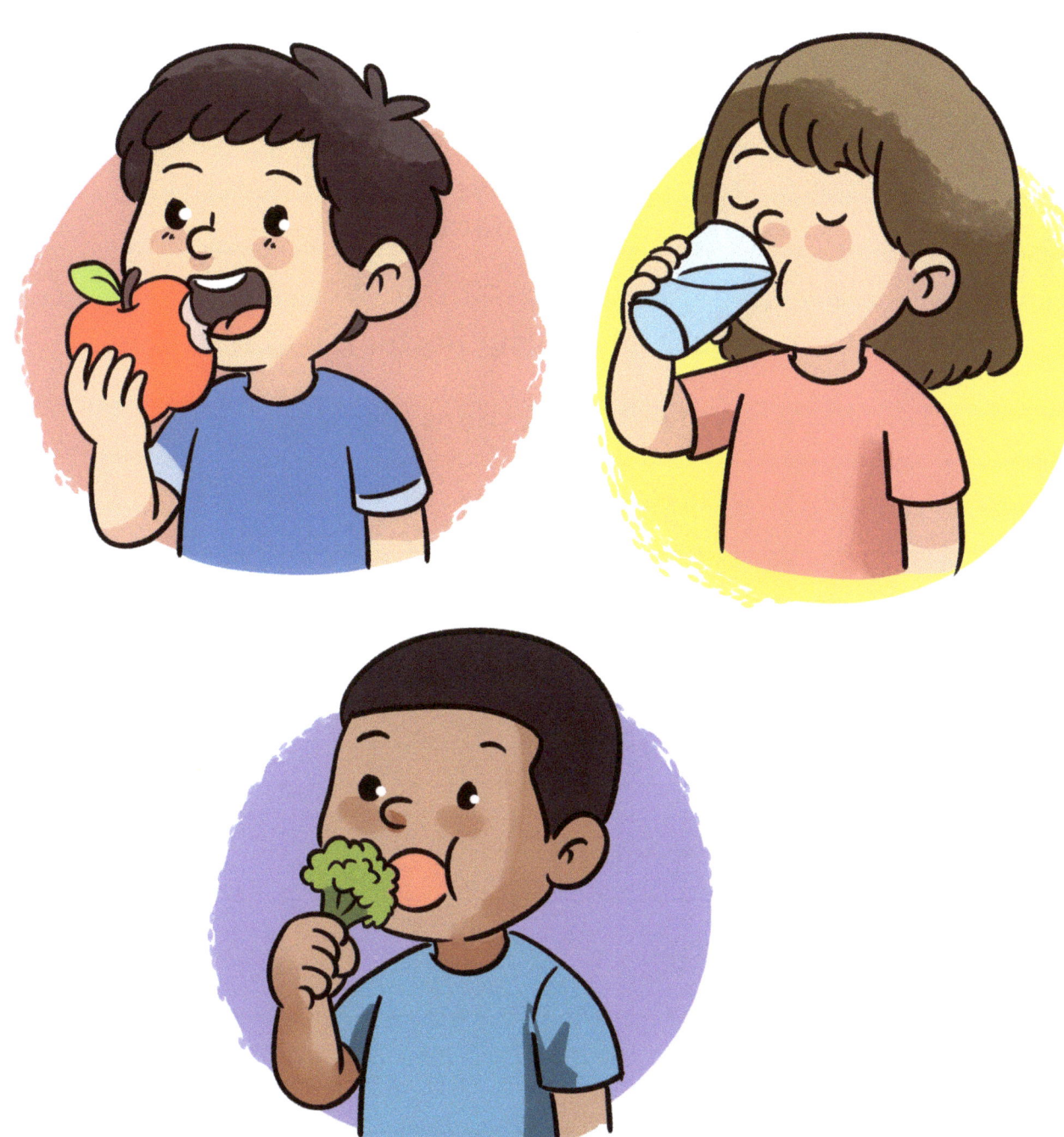

Soon, you will see your doctor to make sure you are healing well and getting stronger.

Your doctor will share ways to help you feel better, get strong, and stay healthy.

If you have any questions, your doctor is happy to help.

Write your questions below.

_____

_____

_____

_____

_____

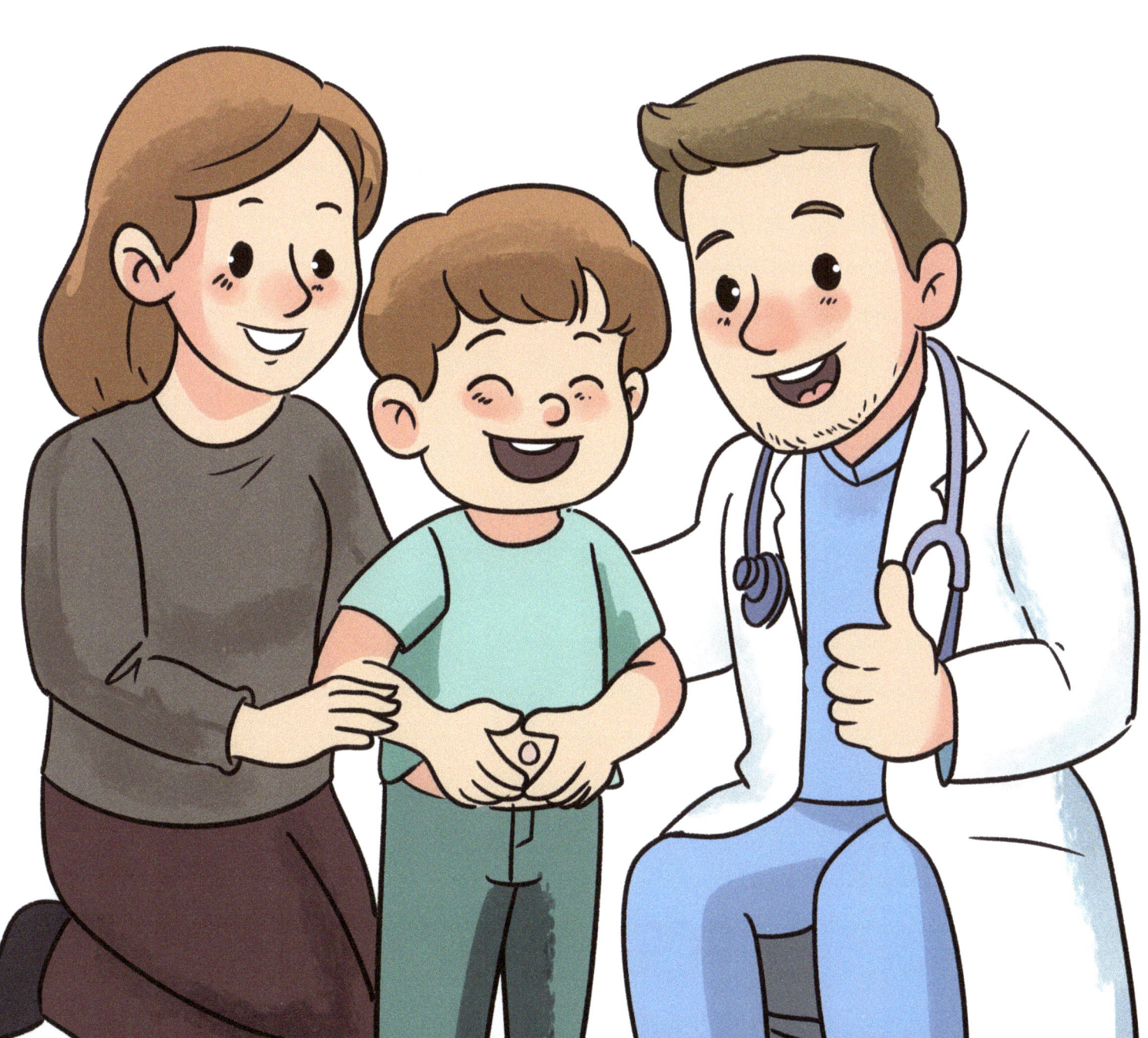

What will you do after your hernia surgery?

A party? A celebration?

What's your favorite way to celebrate?

Draw or write your party plan below.

Speedy recovery!

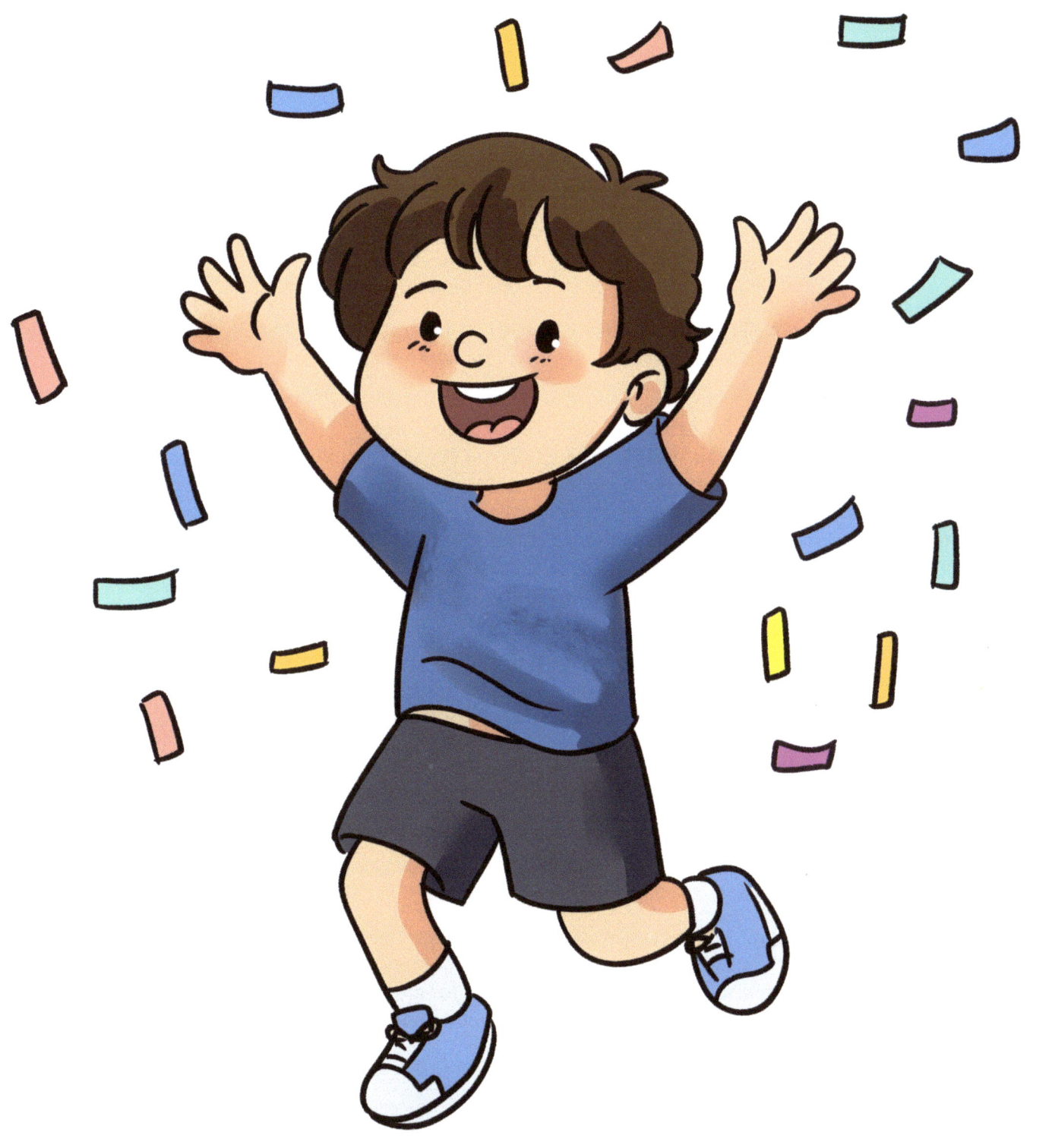

Notes for Parent/Guardian

- If your child's hernia becomes sore, hard, red, swollen, or won't go back in—and especially if they vomit or refuse to eat—it may be an emergency.
Call your child's doctor or go to the ER right away.

- Placement of the intravenous (IV) catheter in this young age group is typically done *after* your child is asleep in the operating room.

- After the surgery, it is common for children to feel confused, disoriented, or irritable, and they may cry, sob, kick, scream, or thrash around.
It normally takes about one hour for the anesthesia to wear off.

- If your little one enjoys daily baths, consider giving them a bath the night before surgery. They may need to wait a few days afterward, since keeping the wound site clean, dry, and free from infection is important for healing.

- Post-surgery instructions/restrictions:
Your child's doctor should give you specific instructions on (1) what your child can and cannot do during the recovery period, (2) the duration of the post-surgical restrictions, and (3) any post-surgical follow-ups. Additionally, (4) they should instruct what to watch out for and when it is necessary for you to bring your child back to the hospital in case of an emergency.
If they forget, please kindly remind them and obtain these instructions/restrictions before leaving the hospital.

Disclaimer

Please note that the illustrations are not drawn to scale.

This book is written for informational, educational, and personal growth purposes and should not be used as a substitute for medical advice.

Please consult your child's doctor if they need medical attention and to ensure the information in this book pertains to your child's medical condition and needs. I cannot guarantee what your child experiences is exactly what is being discussed in this book.

The author and the publisher are not responsible, either directly or indirectly, for any damages, monetary losses, or reparations due to information in this book. By reading this book, the readers agree not to hold the author and the publisher responsible for any losses as a result of any errors, inaccuracies, or omissions in this book.

Please keep in mind that your child's experience depends on the location, the facility, their medical condition, and the healthcare team.
Please use this book in conjunction with your child's doctor's advice. Thank you.

Did this picture book help your child in some way?
If so, I would love to hear about it!

www.amazon.com/gp/product-review/B0FP4GFWML

For other book titles, please visit:

www.fzwbooks.com

Connect with the author

email: books@fzwbooks.com
facebook/instagram: @FZWbooks

Books by the author

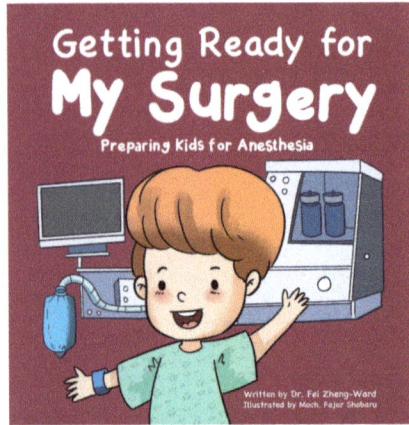 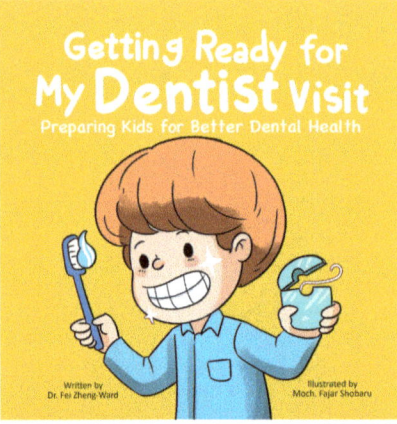 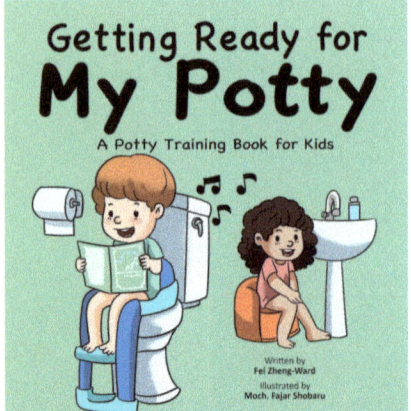
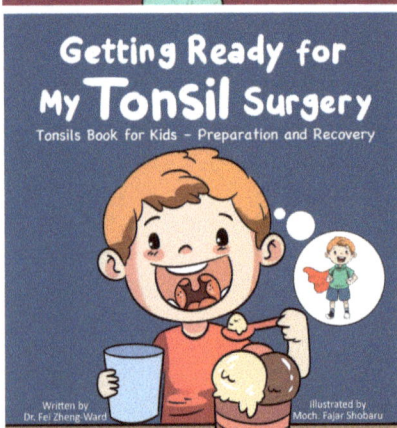 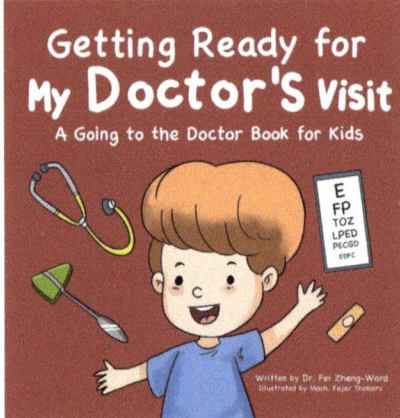 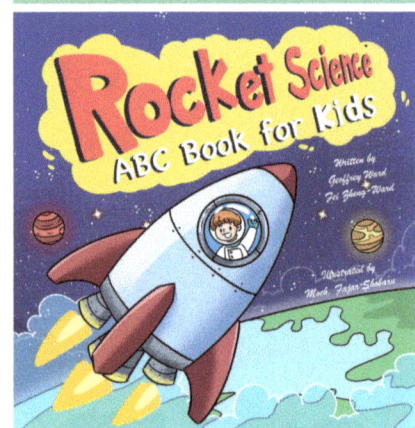
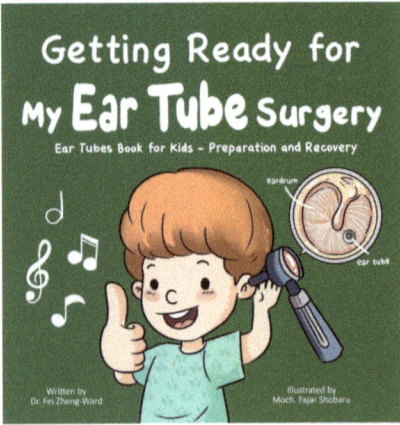 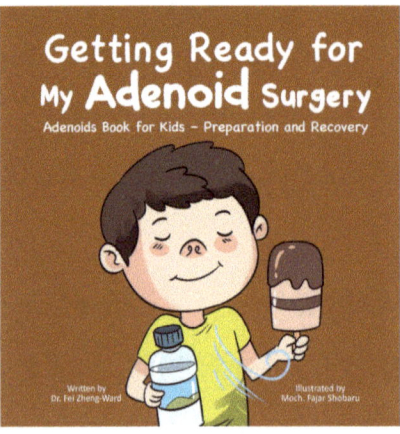 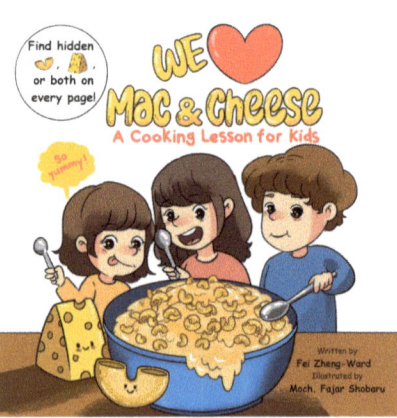

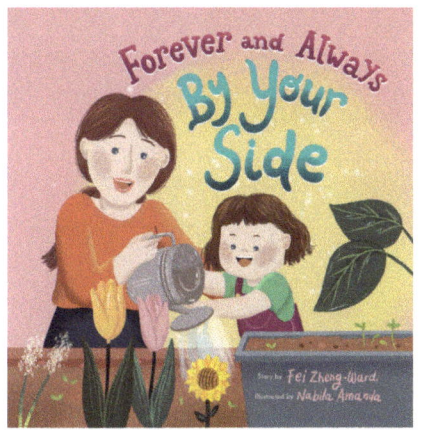
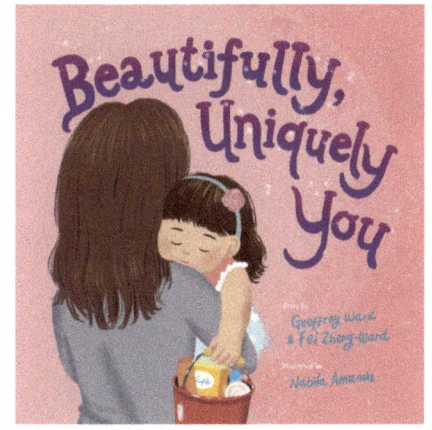
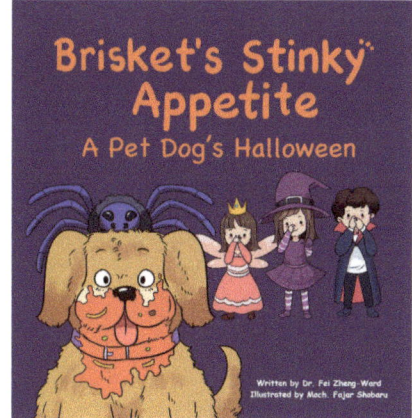
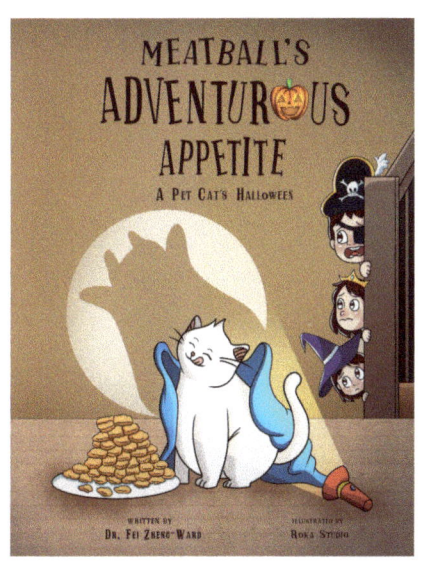
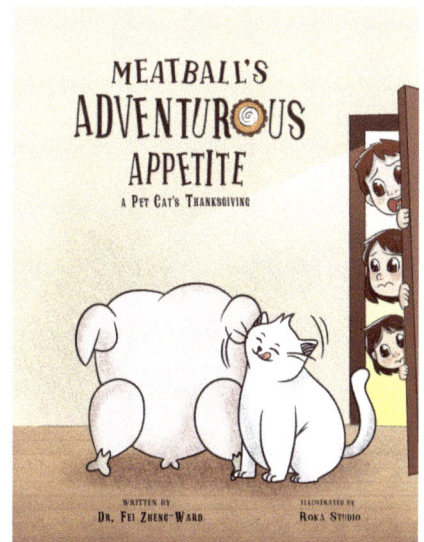
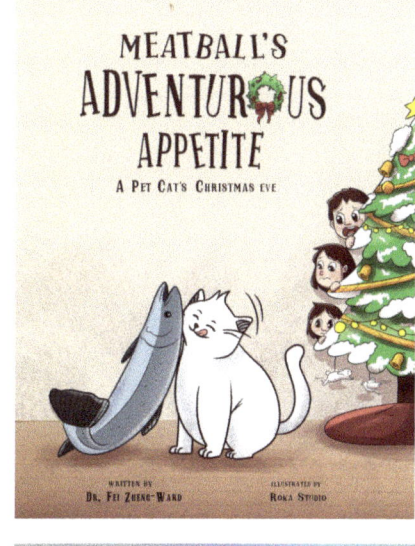
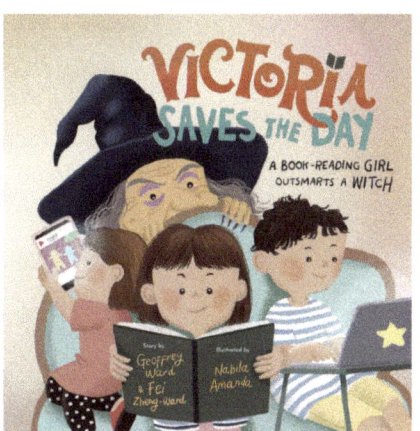
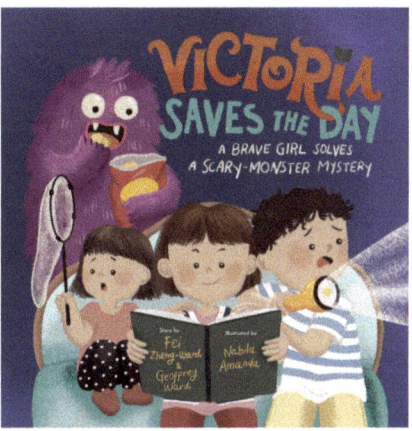
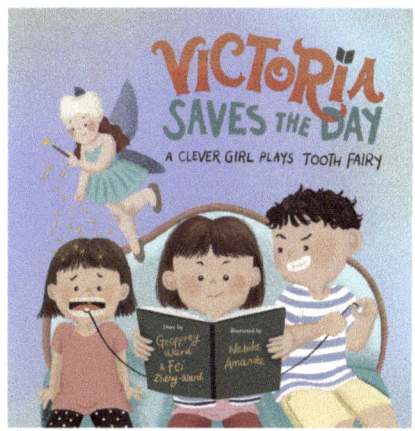

www.ingramcontent.com/pod-product-compliance
Lightning Source LLC
Chambersburg PA
CBHW042359030426

42337CB00032B/5163